FUNCTIONAL
DISORDERS
OF THE FOOT

FUNCTIONAL
DISORDERS OF
THE FOOT

Their Diagnosis and Treatment

BY

FRANK D. DICKSON, M.D., F.A.C.S.

ASSOCIATE PROFESSOR OF CLINICAL SURGERY, MEDICAL SCHOOL,
UNIVERSITY OF KANSAS; ORTHOPEDIC SURGEON, ST. LUKE'S, KANSAS
CITY GENERAL, AND WHEATLEY HOSPITALS, KANSAS CITY, MISSOURI;
PROVIDENCE HOSPITAL, KANSAS CITY, KANSAS

AND

REX L. DIVELEY, A.B., M.D., F.A.C.S

COLONEL, MEDICAL CORPS, ARMY OF THE UNITED STATES;
ORTHOPEDIC CONSULTANT, EUROPEAN THEATER OF OPERATIONS;
ORTHOPEDIC SURGEON, ST. LUKE'S, KANSAS CITY GENERAL,
RESEARCH, AND WHEATLEY HOSPITALS, KANSAS CITY, MISSOURI;
PROVIDENCE HOSPITAL, KANSAS CITY, KANSAS

202 ILLUSTRATIONS

SECOND EDITION

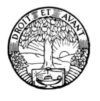

PHILADELPHIA   MONTREAL   LONDON

J. B. LIPPINCOTT COMPANY

PREFACE TO THE SECOND EDITION

In preparing this second edition, no changes have been made in the material dealing with the fundamentals of foot imbalance. Continuing experience has brought to light no evidence which justifies the authors in changing their point of view regarding the fundamental causes of foot imbalance, the manner in which architectural faults and structural weakness give rise to symptom-producing foot disorders, and the effectiveness of the measures advised in relieving symptoms resulting from faulty foot attitudes.

A number of additions have been made to the text. Some of these are for the purpose of clarifying certain points; most of the additions, however, are entirely new material, which it is hoped will add to the completeness of the monograph. A number of additional surgical procedures have been added. These include two additional operations for the correction of flatfoot, one for the correction of hallux varus, and several others dealing with corrections of deformities of the toes.

Two new chapters have been written; one on Functional Disorders of the Foot in Relation to Military Service, and a second on Foot Disorders in Relation to Industry. These additions seemed worthwhile in view of the large numbers in the armed services and employed in industry at this time, a situation which it is felt will continue for some time to come. Functional foot disorders are a real problem, both in military service and in industry, since both require a more extensive use of the feet than is necessary in ordinary peacetime activity.

The chapter on Constitutional Diseases Affecting the Foot has been entirely rewritten. While this subject is too large to be adequately covered in a single chapter, it is hoped that the salient points have been sufficiently emphasized to indicate the importance of constitutional conditions in relation to foot symptoms and to enable a sufficiently accurate diagnosis to be made to insure that adequate treatment will be carried out.

The authors wish to express their sincere thanks to those who have so generously permitted the use of material and illustrations from their published articles. They also desire to acknowledge their indebtedness to Dr. Nicholas S. Pickard for his able assistance in collecting material for the chapter on Constitutional Diseases Affecting the Foot and to their secretary, Emily Carter, for her valuable help in preparing and assembling the material for this edition.

The Authors.

PREFACE TO THE FIRST EDITION

The prevalence of functional foot disorders serious enough to cause definite foot discomfort and disability is recognized generally. It is not commonly appreciated, however, that the interference with comfort and efficiency which results from symptom-producing foot conditions is so widespread as to constitute a problem of considerable economic as well as medical importance. Unfortunately the medical profession as a whole has failed to evaluate correctly the seriousness of disabling foot conditions and consequently has failed to give them the study and attention they deserve. In addition, the public is inclined to look upon foot discomfort as not of sufficient gravity to demand professional advice and the expense of medical treatment, and it follows the most economical course which is self-treatment in the form of purchasing an alleged "corrective" shoe or seeking comparatively inexpensive nonprofessional advice.

As a result, the treatment of functional foot disorders has fallen largely into nonmedical hands. Honest and conscientious as many of those without the medical ranks may be, the fact is true that many of them have not the fundamental training which entitles them to accept the responsibility involved. Because some of these nonmedical groups lack knowledge of the primary causes of disorder and their effect upon the foot, we frequently find that important prophylactic measures are not applied at stages when the greatest benefit is to be derived from their use and that advanced cases of foot disorder are being inadequately treated.

Of the nonmedical groups the chiropodists have made and are making every effort to improve the standards of their schools in many parts of the country so that the graduates may be better trained to meet the demands made upon them.

Many shoe manufacturers are conscientiously striving to produce improved and scientifically sound footwear.

While it is logical to accept trained nonprofessional sources as agencies for disseminating information and help in disorders which are so prevalent as to constitute a public problem—as is the case in functional foot disorders—the fact remains that so long as any of these nonmedical groups is inadequately trained its ability to provide help is rigidly limited and certainly should never extend into the surgical field.

It may be said then that because of lack of interest in foot disorders in the profession and because of lack of fundamental knowledge among the nonmedical groups a very unsatisfactory situation prevails today as regards the management of functional foot disorders. This situation can only be improved by education: education of the profession in the importance of disabling foot conditions; education of the nonmedical groups in the primary causes of foot disorders and their legitimate limitations in carrying out treatment; education of the public to an understanding of the importance of foot welfare.

It is to meet the situation just described, as far as the medical profession is concerned, that this book has been written. It deals chiefly with the clinical aspect of foot disorders. Only such material on the evolutionary development of the foot, on anatomy, and on physiology has been introduced as seemed necessary to an intelligent understanding of the foot as a functioning organ and to an appreciation of those departures from normal which cause painful and incapacitating conditions. Its aim has been to present a practical and perhaps elementary statement of the causes and symptoms of disabling foot conditions and suggest such therapeutic measures as have proved useful in correcting pathology or relieving symptoms.

It has seemed desirable to dwell at some length upon the foot of childhood and adolescence as many of the faults in foot architecture which produce symptoms in the adult have their origin in the growing foot of the child and the developing foot of the adolescent period. As much more can be done to correct architectural faults responsible for the development of functional foot disorders between the ages of two and sixteen years than after the adult age has been reached, this period of foot development seems worthy of careful study. This method of approaching the subject has resulted in a certain amount of repetition in discussing etiology, symptomatology, and treatment, but it seemed best to make each section as complete and self-contained as possible.

Most of the material presented is derived from personal observation and experience, but the authors have not hesitated to quote from the work of others. Credit has been given in every instance to those whose material has been used, so far as this is known; if credit has not been given, it is an oversight for which the authors sincerely apologize.

Frank D. Dickson, M.D.

Rex L. Diveley, M.D.

CONTENTS

xi

EVOLUTIONARY DEVELOPMENT OF THE HUMAN FOOT

The human foot represents the sum of innumerable changes in form and structure which have taken place during its evolutionary history. This evolutionary history began with the appearance of primitive vertebrate limbs and progressed through the amphibian, reptilian, mammalian, and early primate periods to the present human form. During all the centuries of development through which the foot has passed, it has changed in architecture and function to meet the demands placed upon it as locomotion became more and more extensive and complicated. These demands reached their culmination when the upright position was assumed, and the entire responsibility of the support of the body was thrust upon the foot. Obviously then, an understanding of the normal anatomy and physiology of the human foot as it is today can be reached only through an insight into its evolutionary background.

There is at the present time considerable difference of opinion among authorities as to the factors which were responsible for the changes in structure and architecture of the foot during its evolutionary history. There are those who believe from their investigations that muscle action was responsible for these changes, and that it was function rather than form which brought about the sequence of modifications which resulted in the human foot; this group is comprised of Sir Arthur Keith and his followers. There are others who believe that these changes were the result of both external and internal factors—the action of gravity plus the propulsive effort of muscles—which are complementary to each other; this is the view of Dr. Dudley Morton. While these two groups differ as to the pathway along which the evolution of the foot has progressed, they are in agreement as to the modifications which have taken place and on the characteristics of normal structure and function of the human foot as it is today.

It is impossible in a monograph of this type to deal extensively with foot evolution and to discuss the various anthropological theories of foot development which have been advanced from time to time. The views on foot evolution presented by Dr. Dudley J. Morton in *The Journal of Bone and Joint Surgery*, for January and March, 1924, and later in his book, *The Human Foot*, have been selected as the basis for the brief discussion of foot evolution presented here. The reason for the selection lies in the belief that his studies are the most recent, the most exhaustive, and certainly the most convincing with which the authors are familiar. That the views of Sir Arthur Keith, who has made a careful study of the foot from the anthropological standpoint, deserve equal rating with those of Morton is not disputed, but it seems unwise to complicate this text by attempting to analyze and compare the different theories of foot evolution. This brief chapter on the evolution of the human foot is intended only to outline in a very sketchy manner, as a desirable prelude to the study of functional disorders of the foot, the important changes in structure and architecture through which the foot has passed in its centuries of development; it does not pretend to discuss foot evolution in detail nor to offer any original views on foot development. Those who wish to pursue the study of foot evolution or who are desirous of determining for themselves the forces which are responsible for moulding the human foot to its present form, will find the writings of Sir Arthur Keith, Dr. Dudley Morton, and others most interesting and instructive.

ARBOREAL LIFE

The origin of primate life took place in the trees. Our ancestors were of arboreal stock and the foot was used for grasping purposes. The type of foot best adapted to such use was one in which the fore or the grasping part of the foot was highly developed, flexible, and strong; the heel which rested but lightly on the supporting branch was unimportant, little used, and rudimentary. The arboreal foot then is characterized by long, flexible phalanges and metatarsal bones, a small medially projecting hallux resembling a thumb in form and action, and a rudimentary heel which does not contact the ground (Fig. 1). In this type of foot, there is a definite degree of supination or turning inward of the forepart of the foot so that the inner or medial side of the foot is concave, and the lateral or outer side of the foot convex; it resembles in

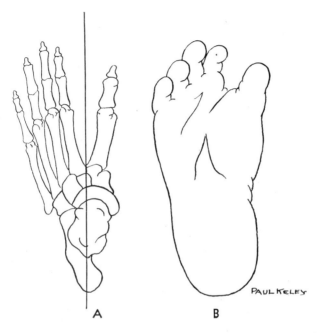

FIG. 1. Primate feet. A, the bones and location of the functional axis of the foot in the gorilla; B, plantar aspect of the foot of a mountain gorilla. (From D. J. Morton.)

form, though not in behavior, a congenital club foot. When such an arboreal foot was placed upon a flat surface, the ground, the outer border first came in contact with the weight-bearing surface. However, as the body weight in the upright position falls toward the medial border of the foot and as the arboreal foot was an extremely flexible one, the medial border depressed under the burden of the superimposed weight until it also came in contact with the ground and the foot became flat. This is what probably occurred as our ancestors forsook arboreal life and through gradual gradations became terrestrial.

TERRESTRIAL LIFE

The demands of terrestrial life were quite different from those of arboreal life and these changed demands necessitated certain changes in the architecture of the foot in order that they might be successfully met.

One of the first important alterations in architecture demanded by terrestrial life was a change in the shape of the foot to provide a firm, reliable base of support because of the habitual assumption of the erect position. To provide this there occurred, through

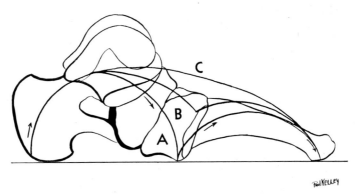

Fig. 2. Lateral view of arboreal foot on a flat surface (hallux removed to give better view). A, the early double arc due to contact of the cuneiform bone with the ground; B, the broken arc which indicates the direction of the line of movement of force when contact of the cuneiform bone with the ground is broken; C, the natural line which the forces of leverage would follow when the metatarsal heads act as a fulcrum. (From D. J. Morton.)

contact with the ground, a marked development of the rudimentary heel to prevent tipping backward; forward tipping was already provided against by the well-developed forepart of the foot. In the human foot, then, a weight-bearing heel developed through gradual transition and became the posterior point of weight bearing.

The second important alteration in architecture was brought about by a change in the function of the foot to meet another important demand of terrestrial life; it ceased to be a grasping organ and became an organ of locomotion. Leverage was necessary for propulsion in locomotion, and the flat, arboreal foot was poorly adapted for leverage action since this act was performed on a short anterior lever arm composed of the metatarsal bones; the depressed internal cuneiform bone (Fig. 2), which had come to lie in contact with the ground through descent of the arboreal foot, acted as the fulcrum. In such a prehuman foot, locomotion

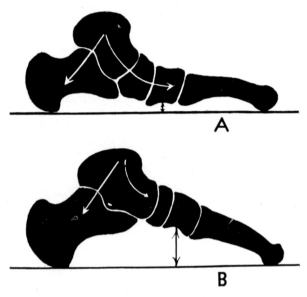

Fig. 3. A, lateral view of arboreal foot showing arrangement of bones and weight stresses; B, same view of human foot showing the elevation of the scaphoid and internal cuneiform and weight stresses. (From D. J. Morton.)

would, by reason of the short lever arm, throw a severe strain on the metatarsal bones and joints, and the body weight in walking would be rapidly shifted from one foot to the other to lessen the strain. Progression in the prehuman foot was accomplished by a shift of the body weight from one foot to the other, rather than by a leverage action of the foot itself; and the gait was a side to side swaying, a method of progress which resembles that of a person with a very bad flat foot. The demand for rapid and extensive movement was one of the necessities of terrestrial life, and improvement in the mechanics of the foot through evolutionary modifications to enhance its leverage and propulsive action would certainly progress with the utmost rapidity. Briefly, this improvement took the form of a gradual elevation from the ground of the internal cuneiform and scaphoid bones through the development of strong plantar ligaments and the action of the leg muscles, which gradually increased in strength and importance under the demands made upon them (Fig. 3). As the scaphoid and internal cuneiform bones were raised from the ground, they ceased to be the fulcrum of the propulsive lever and this duty was shifted to the heads of the metatarsal bones, particularly the first and second metatarsals, which became the anterior pier of the inner longitudinal arch which developed as the scaphoid and cuneiform bones were elevated.

Coincident with the elevation of the scaphoid and cuneiform bones, there occurred a change in the form and position of the os calcis which was of the greatest importance. In the arboreal foot, the inclination of the superior surface of the os calcis is strongly downward and inward. The facets on its superior surface, which receive the astragalus, have the same inclination; consequently, in the arboreal foot as the body weight is received by the astragalus, these facets tend, by their inclination, to direct the greater part of the load toward the medial or inner side of the foot. During the course of evolution, as the scaphoid and cuneiform bones were gradually elevated, the anterior part of the os calcis was elevated along with them, probably largely through pressure of the tendons of the leg muscles passing under the sustentaculum tali. As the anterior part of the os calcis was raised, it carried with it the cuboid bone and an outer longitudinal arch was formed (Fig. 4). In addition, as its forepart was elevated, the entire os calcis rotated outward; and as this rotation occurred, the facets on its superior surface, instead of looking inward and downward, faced forward, downward, and only slightly inward (Figs. 4 and 5). This change in the position of the facets of the os calcis resulted in shifting the major part of the body weight toward the lateral side of the foot, which gradually became a more important functioning part. To meet the demands of increased weight stresses, there took place a gradual development of the outer metatarsal bones of which the fifth metatarsal eventually became the anterior pillar of the outer, or short, longitudinal arch. The tuberosity of

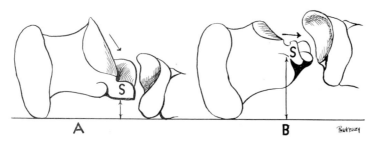

FIG. 4. Oblique posterior-inner lateral view of chimpanzee (A) and human (B) calcaneal and scaphoid bones, showing the respective positions of the sustentaculum tali (S), in the arboreal (A) and human (B) foot under superimposed weight. The arrows above the facets indicate the direction of their inclination which, in the arboreal foot (A), is abruptly downward and inward, and in the human foot (B) more directly forward. (From D. J. Morton.)

the os calcis, by reason of its development and the elevation of the anterior part of this bone, became the posterior point of con-

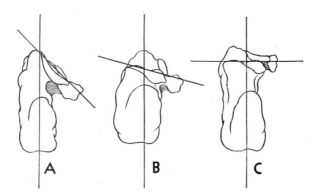

FIG. 5. Posterior view of the left calcanea of the gorilla (A), Neanderthal man (B), and modern man (C), showing the strong inward slant of the subtalar joint surface in the gorilla foot, its modified slant in Neanderthal man, and only a mild retention of that slant in the modern human foot. (From D. J. Morton.)

tact between the foot and the ground and so came to form the posterior pier of both the internal and the external longitudinal arches.

The third important change had to do with alteration in the hallux. In the arboreal foot the hallux, and its metatarsal bone, was long and slender, had a marked divergence inward so that it was widely separated from the second metatarsal and its digit and was extremely mobile. The hallux in the arboreal foot resembled a thumb in form and function. As life on the ground was adopted, the divergent position of the hallux at first persisted as an efficient

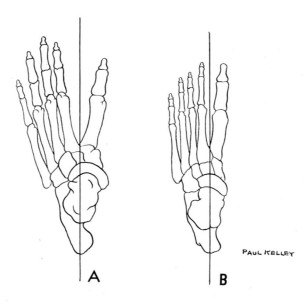

PAUL KELLEY

A   B

Fig. 6. Bones and line of functional axis in the foot of the gorilla, A; in the human foot, B. (From D. J. Morton.)

support against the strong inward deflection of the body weight due to the inclination downward and inward of the superior surface of the calcaneum. However, as the body weight was distributed more and more on the lateral portion of the foot, the inward divergence of the hallux decreased and the first metatarsal and hallux became more nearly parallel to the second metatarsal and its digit, and less mobile. This change in the position and mobility of the first metatarsal bone comprised a definite improvement in the foot as a weight-bearing organ because it brought about a more compact arrangement of the bones of the forefoot.

In addition, as this change brought the anterior and posterior halves of the foot into alignment, its leverage and propulsive action were improved (Fig. 6).

Finally, as the leverage action of the foot necessary to locomotion on the ground demanded structural rigidity in the foot, the plantar ligaments became more important and increased in strength to give this added rigidity. As the ligaments became stronger the intrinsic muscles of the foot, so important in the grasping foot, became smaller and less important.

SUMMARY

We have, as the result of its adaption to the needs of terrestrial life, three characteristics developing in the human foot: (1) It became plantigrade through the development of the heel to meet the needs of the upright position for an anterior-posterior base of support. (2) It became more compact in order to sustain the burden placed upon it by the assumption of the fully upright position. (3) It underwent changes in the form and arrangement of its individual bones to meet the demands of leverage action necessary for efficient locomotion on the ground. These latter changes resulted in the formation of two longitudinal arches, a long inner arch formed by the tuberosity of the os calcis, the astragalus, the scaphoid, the cuneiform and the first and second metatarsal bones, and a short outer longitudinal arch formed by the tuberosity of the os calcis, the cuboid, and the fifth metatarsal bones. With such extensive evolutionary changes taking place, it is possible that even today the work is not complete or at least the pattern not so firmly established that faulty casts may not be turned out by the mould. It is understandable, in other words, that the foot of an individual may fail, in detail, to complete all of the evolutionary changes necessary for the successful performance of its function as an organ of support and locomotion; it may fall short of the standard design and display weaknesses of form and structure which doom it to the role of a weakling and so unable to function as it should under the stress of use.

2

ANATOMY

A knowledge of the structure of the normal foot is essential to an intelligent appreciation of such departures from normal as are encountered in it from time to time. Some discussion of the normal anatomy of the foot then is a necessary prelude to a study of foot disorders, the basis of which is usually some distortion or variation of the foot's normal anatomic arrangement. It does not seem necessary to repeat here the extensive descriptive anatomy of the foot to be found in any textbook of anatomy, and only such features of its anatomy will be considered as are necessary to an intelligent understanding of the foot as a functioning organ. Since there is a difference of opinion among authorities regarding some of the details of the anatomy of the foot, many of the statements to follow may differ with opinions expressed elsewhere. The views here expressed, however, seem to be those most generally accepted as far as can be determined.

BONES OF THE FOOT

The foot is made up of a combination of twenty-six bones; seven tarsal bones, five metatarsals, and fourteen phalanges. The tarsal bones are the astragalus, os calcis, scaphoid or navicular, cuboid, internal, middle, and external cuneiform. Anteriorly, the tarsals articulate with the five metatarsals. The fourteen phalanges extend forward from the metatarsals, three in each of the second, third, fourth, and fifth toes, and two in the first or great toe (Figs. 7-8).

Tarsal Bones

The astragalus, a wedge-shaped bone, fits into the mortice formed by the distal ends of the tibia and fibula and, together with these bones, forms the ankle joint. Below, the body of the astragalus articulates loosely with the os calcis or heel bone to form the posterior part of the subastragalar joint. Anteriorly, the head of the astragalus extends forward and slightly inward to articulate with the scaphoid and to form the anterior portion of the subastragalar joint.

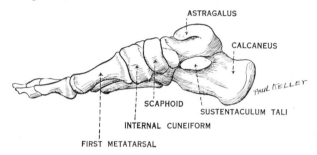

ASTRAGALUS

CALCANEUS

SCAPHOID

SUSTENTACULUM TALI

INTERNAL CUNEIFORM

FIRST METATARSAL

Fig. 7. Bone structure of the foot, medial aspect. (Redrawn after Davis, Applied Anatomy, J. B. Lippincott Co.)

The os calcis is the largest bone in the foot. It is narrow and elongated, forms the heel, supports the astragalus, and articulates with the cuboid in front. It has six surfaces, of which the inferior, medial, and superior are important. At the back or posterior part the inferior surface presents an enlargement or tuberosity divided

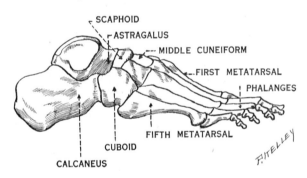

SCAPHOID

ASTRAGALUS

MIDDLE CUNEIFORM

FIRST METATARSAL

PHALANGES

FIFTH METATARSAL

CUBOID

CALCANEUS

Fig. 8. Bone structure of the foot, lateral aspect. (Redrawn after Davis, Applied Anatomy, J. B. Lippincott Co.)

into the internal and external tubercles. This tuberosity forms the posterior pier or weight-bearing surface of the foot. A shelf-like process, the sustentaculum tali, which serves as a support for the head of the astragalus is at the front and projects inward from the medial surface. The superior surface carries two facets: one, posterior, which articulates with the inferior surface of the body of the astragalus; and one, anterior, on the sustentaculum tali which articulates with the inferior surface of the head of the astragalus.

The cuboid, a small square bone, articulates with the os calcis behind, with the proximal ends of the outer two metatarsals in front and with the scaphoid and external cuneiform on its medial side.

The scaphoid is a disc-shaped bone, concave posteriorly and convex anteriorly. It articulates with the astragalus posteriorly, with the three cuneiform bones anteriorly, and with the cuboid laterally. The scaphoid bone forms the apex of the long arch of the foot and bears a great mechanical strain.

The three cuneiform bones, internal, middle, and external, articulate with the scaphoid posteriorly to form the medial portion of the midtarsal joint and anteriorly with the inner three metatarsals.

Metatarsals and Phalanges

There are five metatarsal bones. The first metatarsal bone is the largest; the other four are approximately of equal size. The first three metatarsal bones articulate with the cuneiform bones and the outer two with the cuboid.

There are two phalanges in the great toe and three each in the remaining toes, known as the proximal, middle, and distal phalanges.

Located beneath the head of the first metatarsal are two small sesamoid bones, which lie in the tendon of the flexor brevis hallucis muscle. At times a small sesamoid is found under the interphalangeal joint of the great toe. Occasionally, one is found under the metatarsophalangeal joint of the second and fifth toes and more rarely beneath the third and fourth (Fig. 9).

Foot Proper

The seven tarsal and the five metatarsal bones comprise the foot proper. Through these bones the body weight is transmitted to the weight-bearing surface, and any abnormality of these bones or any variation in their normal alignment with each other will alter the architecture of the foot and in all probability interfere with its proper use.

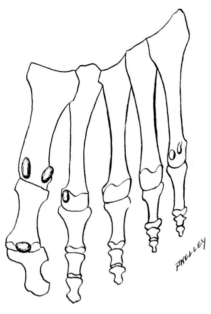

FIG. 9. Position and location of the sesamoid bones of the foot. (Redrawn after Davis, Applied Anatomy, J. B. Lippincott Co.)

LIGAMENTS OF THE FOOT

Since strength is necessary in an organ which must support the entire body weight, the bones of the foot are bound together by strong and numerous ligaments. The most important of these, as far as concerns this study, are:

1. The internal lateral ligament of the ankle.
2. The external lateral ligament of the ankle.
3. The posterior tibiotarsal ligament of the ankle.
4. The inferior calcaneoscaphoid ligament.
5. The long calcaneocuboid ligament.
6. The plantar fascia.

The internal lateral ligament is attached above to the internal malleolus and divides, as it passes downward, into three distinct strands. The anterior passes forward and inserts into the scaphoid bone and the calcaneoscaphoid ligament. The middle fibers insert into the astragalus and the sustentaculum tali of the os calcis. The posterior strand passes backward and inserts into the astragalus (Fig. 10).

The external lateral ligament is composed of three distinct strands, all attached to the external malleolus. The anterior fibers

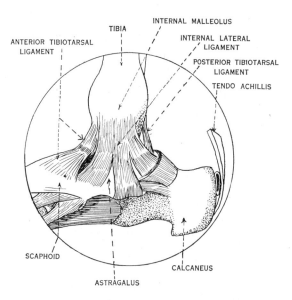

Fig. 10. Ligaments on the medial aspect of the ankle and foot. (Redrawn after Davis, Applied Anatomy, J. B. Lippincott Co.)

run forward and attach to the astragalus. The middle strand passes directly downward and inserts into the lateral surface of the os calcis. The posterior fibers pass backward and insert into the tubercle on the posterior surface of the astragalus (Fig. 11).

These ligaments are most important as they aid in maintaining the stability and lateral balance of the ankle and subastragalar joints.

The posterior tibiotarsal ligament of the ankle joint is a thin, broad band which passes downward from the posterior margin of the articular surface of the tibia, and inserts into the posterior

lower surface of the astragalus behind its trochlear surface. This
ligamentous band acts as a check to extreme dorsal flexion of the
foot and aids in maintaining the anterior-posterior balance of
the foot on the leg (Fig. 11).

The inferior calcaneoscaphoid ligament is an exceedingly
thick and strong band which is attached posteriorly to the anterior
margin of the sustentaculum tali of the os calcis and passes forward and inward to attach to the under surface of the scaphoid
bone. This band supplies a strong support to the head of the

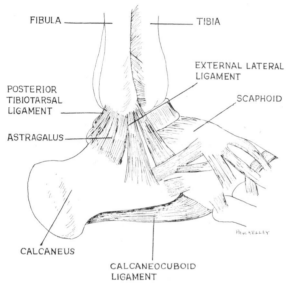

FIBULA _____   _____ TIBIA

EXTERNAL LATERAL
LIGAMENT

POSTERIOR
TIBIOTARSAL
LIGAMENT

SCAPHOID

ASTRAGALUS

CALCANEUS

CALCANEOCUBOID
LIGAMENT

Fig. 11. Ligaments on the lateral aspect of the ankle and foot. (Redrawn after
Davis, Applied Anatomy, J. B. Lippincott Co.)

astragalus and aids in maintaining the integrity of the long arch
of the foot (Fig. 12).

The long calcaneocuboid or plantar ligament is attached
posteriorly to the under surface of the os calcis and runs forward to attach to the inferior surface of the cuboid and bases
of the second, third, fourth and fifth metatarsal bones (Fig.
12).

The plantar fascia, while not a true ligament, functions as a
ligament, and is one of the most important structures of the

foot. It is attached posteriorly to the internal and external tubercles of the os calcis (posterior pillars of the longitudinal arches), and runs forward to attach to the sides of the metatarsophalangeal articulations and the bases of the proximal phalanges. This heavy.

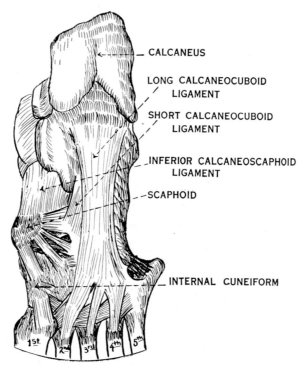

CALCANEUS

LONG CALCANEOCUBOID
LIGAMENT

SHORT CALCANEOCUBOID
LIGAMENT

INFERIOR CALCANEOSCAPHOID
LIGAMENT

SCAPHOID

INTERNAL CUNEIFORM

1st. 2nd 3rd 4th 5th

FIG. 12. Ligaments on the sole of the foot. (Redrawn after Davis, Applied Anat omy, J. B. Lippincott Co.)

strong, triangular band as it spans the pillars of the longitudinal arches, acts as a bow string and aids in maintaining the long arches in their proper positions (Fig. 13).

The numerous short dorsal, plantar, and transverse ligaments are all important elements in the architecture of the foot. It is felt, however, that no useful purpose would be served by entering into a detailed discussion of these minor ligaments; it should suffice to say that each has a place in that very complicated and fairly efficient mechanism, the foot.

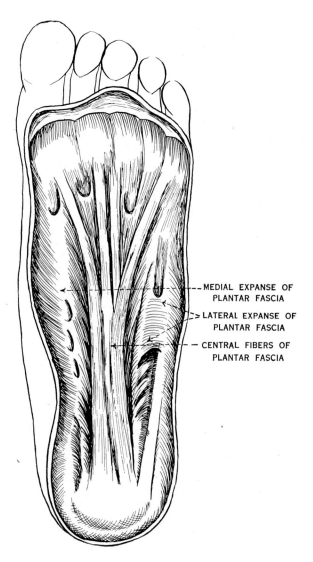

MEDIAL EXPANSE OF
PLANTAR FASCIA

LATERAL EXPANSE OF
PLANTAR FASCIA

CENTRAL FIBERS OF
PLANTAR FASCIA

FIG. 13. Plantar fascia.

JOINTS OF THE FOOT

Between the bones which comprise the foot lie joints which give to it the qualities of flexibility and adaptability. The joints of the phalanges naturally permit the considerable mobility necessary to the proper functioning of these appendages; they

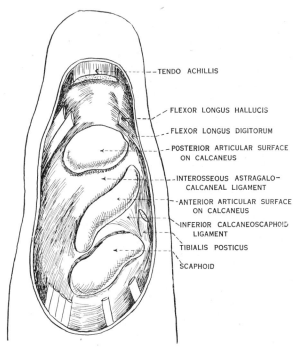

FIG. 14. The lower surface of the subastragalar joint. The astragalus has been removed.

have no special features which require discussion. The joints that lie between the bones which comprise the foot proper permit but a slight gliding movement except the subastragalar joint which has a rather wide range of mobility and deserves special discussion.

The subastragalar joint (Fig. 14) is composed of the articulating surfaces of the astragalus, os calcis, and scaphoid bones, and the calcaneo-astragaloid ligament. This articulation is divided into a posterior part, the calcaneo-astragalar joint, and an anterior part, the calcaneoscapho-astragalar joint.

THE CALCANEO-ASTRAGALAR joint is formed by the posterior facet of the superior surface of the os calcis and the inferior surface of the body of the astragalus.

THE CALCANEOSCAPHO-ASTRAGALAR joint is formed by the anterior facet on the superior surface of the os calcis, which lies on that medially projecting part of the os calcis called the sustentaculum tali, the inferior calcaneoscaphoid ligament, the scaphoid, and the head of the astragalus. The motions in these two joints occur together, and, since it resembles in its construction a ball-and-socket joint, the range of motion permitted is considerable. Most of the lateral and rotary movements possible in the foot occur in this joint.

The action of the joints as related to the function of the foot will be discussed in the chapter on physiology.

ARCHES OF THE FOOT

The arches of the foot are so intimately associated in the minds of most students with the bones of the foot that a description of these arches naturally follows the discussion of the individual foot bones. Today any conception of the arches of the foot put forward must necessarily be a composite one, since so many different views are held concerning the architecture and mechanics of these arches. The authors have chosen to use as a basis for the discussion of the functional disorders of the foot which is to follow that conception of the arches of the foot most generally accepted at this time. Dudley Morton in his recently published book, *The Human Foot*, has expressed views on the architecture of the foot which are decidedly at variance with any hitherto proposed and has supported his claims with most important evidence brought out through extensive studies of the evolution of the human foot. That Morton's work rationalizes many hitherto inadequately explained causes of foot imbalance can not be denied; nevertheless, in a monograph of this type it seems best for purposes of simplicity and clarity to adhere to the commonly accepted conception of the architecture of the foot. Morton's work, however, seems so important that, in as far as is possible, without interfering with the continuity of the subject matter, his views will be commented upon when they seem to have a direct bearing on the subject under discussion.

Of the twenty-six bones which comprise the skeleton of the foot, twelve form the tarsus and metatarsus, and fourteen provide the frame work for the toes. For purposes of clarity it seems best to separate the foot into the foot proper, composed of the tarsus and metatarsus, and the appendages or toes. The reason for this lies in the fact that only the bones of the tarsus and metatarsus enter into the formation of the arches of the foot. The phalanges, while of the greatest importance in the functioning of the foot as a whole, may be ignored as far as the arches are concerned.

The twelve bones of the foot proper are so arranged as to form structural devices known as arches. The arch form of structural arrangement has two advantages: It is mechanically strong and at the same time possesses the quality of resilience which carries with it the ability to absorb shocks and to impart elasticity in action. The structural design of the arches of the foot has been described in a number of different forms by various writers, but the simplest conception, and therefore the best for practical purposes, is that which considers that we have in the foot a longitudinal arch which extends from the heel forward to the heads of the metatarsal bones, and a transverse metatarsal arch which extends across the front of the foot from the head of the first metatarsal to the head of the fifth metatarsal.

The longitudinal arch is usually separated into an inner or long longitudinal arch, and an outer or short longitudinal arch. The inner longitudinal arch is formed by the os calcis, astragalus, scaphoid, cuneiform and the first, second, and third metatarsal bones (Fig. 15). The outer longitudinal arch is formed by the os calcis, the cuboid, and the fourth and fifth metatarsal bones (Fig. 16). It will be observed that with this conception of the structure of the longitudinal arch of the foot, both longitudinal arches converge posteriorly at the os calcis, and make contact with the bearing surface through the tuberosity of the os calcis. The tuberosity of the os calcis then forms the posterior pier of both internal and external longitudinal arches. As they pass forward, the longitudinal arches diverge so that the inner longitudinal arch makes contact with the bearing surface through the head of the first metatarsal, which may be looked upon as its anterior pier; and the outer longitudinal arch, through the head of the fifth metatarsal bone which forms its anterior pier.

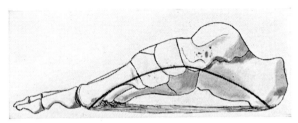

Fig. 15. Bone structure of the foot from the medial side showing the plantar fascia and the construction of the long longitudinal arch.

The transverse or metatarsal arch, as it is commonly accepted, is formed by the heads of the five metatarsals (Fig. 17). With this conception of a metatarsal arch, the head of the first metatarsal forms the inner pier of the arch, the fifth metatarsal head, the

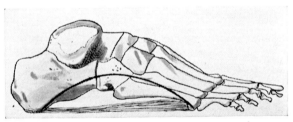

Fig. 16. Bone structure of the foot from the lateral side showing the plantar fascia and the construction of the short or lateral longitudinal arch.

outer pier, and the remaining three metatarsal heads form a slightly dorsally convex bridge between. The metatarsal heads, while ordinarily quite movable on each other, are held firmly in an arch formation by the transverse ligament and supporting muscles.

WEIGHT-BEARING

With such an arrangement of a double longitudinal arch, extending from the heel forward, and an anteriorly placed transverse arch, it is evident that the foot, as a whole, does not make contact with the bearing surface but that we have in the foot a three-point bearing through which the body weight rests upon the ground. The three points of bearing, or contact, are the tuberosity of the os calcis posteriorly and the heads of the first and fifth meta-

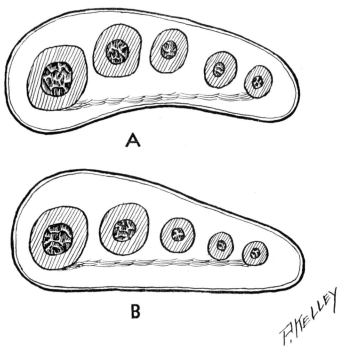

FIG. 17. A transverse section of the foot through the metatarsal region showing the transverse fascia. A, normal metatarsal arch; B, fallen or depressed metatarsal arch.

tarsal bones anteriorly (Fig. 18). The body weight is received by the astragalus and by it is transmitted to the three-point contact through the arches. It is the resiliency and elasticity inherent in this structural arrangement which enables the foot to sustain the body weight with a minimum of strain, cushion impacts which result from certain forms of activity, and give spring to the gait in walking, running, jumping, etc.

While the above described arrangement of the arches is the one

most generally held at this time, it should be stated that there
are many who deny that there is a transverse metatarsal arch, and
there is some disagreement as to the exact form which the longitudinal arches take. While it would not be desirable to attempt
to discuss all of the ideas regarding the architecture of the foot

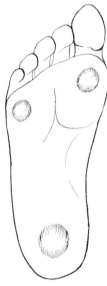

FIG. 18. The three principal weight-bearing points on the normal foot.

which differ from that stated above, it does seem worthwhile at
this point briefly to discuss the conclusions which Dudley J.
Morton has recently published.

In its essentials, Morton's theory of the architecture of the foot
has two major premises as follows: (1) That instead of being considered as a single unit, the foot should be divided into five individual arcs or arches, conforming to its metatarsal bones. These
arcs converge at the heel posteriorly and extend to the head of
each of the five metatarsal bones anteriorly. (2) That while there
is a transverse midtarsal arch made up of three cuneiform bones,
the cuboid bone, and the base of the fifth metatarsal bone, a
transverse metatarsal arch, composed of the heads of the metatarsals, does not exist. He bases his opinion of the absence of the

metatarsal arch upon evidence secured by examination of one hundred and fifty individuals, using an instrument called a statocometer to measure the weight distribution in various parts of the foot. The statocometer is so designed that through three plates upon which the foot rests (one for the heel and two for the forepart of the foot) the weight borne by each metatarsal head can be determined. The observations made by Morton with the statocometer showed that not only did the head of each metatarsal bone have contact with the bearing surface but also that each shared equally in the support of the body weight with the exception of Metatarsal I which bore a double share. Morton, therefore, assumed that there is no transverse metatarsal arch formed by the heads of the metatarsal bones. The conclusion which Morton has arrived at in regard to the weight-bearing of the heads of the metatarsal bones seems to have some importance in indicating the underlying cause of certain types of functional foot disorders. It will be referred to later when these conditions are under discussion.

Lake expressed the opinion that the presence of an anterior or metatarsal arch is not incompatible with the fact that the heads of the metatarsal bones are all in contact with the ground. He reasons that, since the metatarsal bones are relatively of varying length because of the architecture of the foot, with the presence of an arch they might all reach and lie in contact with the ground. Even so, he feels that this arch is unimportant anatomically.

Notwithstanding the doubt as to the presence of a metatarsal arch which has been expressed by a number of investigators the concept that such a metatarsal arch does exist is widely held. Because of the general acceptance of such an arch and because so many functional ailments of the foot affect the metatarsal region, it seems best to retain for the present at least the theory of a metatarsal arch as part of the structure of the foot.

MUSCLES AND TENDONS OF THE FOOT

The muscles of the foot are important, for they perform three very necessary functions: That of carrying out the movements in the foot required for locomotion; that of maintaining the leg in a balanced position over the foot (postural stability); and that of serving as supports to the arches of the foot. The muscles of the foot include those which lie in the leg and send tendons into the foot, usually called the long muscles, and those which lie entirely within the foot, the short or intrinsic muscles.

Long Muscles

The long muscles of the foot, in as far as they impart movement to the foot, may be divided into four groups: Those which dorsally flex or raise the foot from the ground—the tibialis anticus and the peroneus tertius, acting together, the extensor longus digitorum, and the extensor longus hallucis (Fig. 19). Those which plantar flex the foot, lift the heel and propel the body when taking a step— the soleus, gastrocnemius, flexor longus digitorum, and the flexor longus hallucis (Fig. 20). The adductors or those which draw the foot inward into inversion—the tibialis posticus and tibialis anticus (Fig. 21). The abductors evert the foot or draw it outward—the peroneus longus, peroneus brevis, and peroneus tertius (Fig. 19). It is largely through the action of the long muscles that the various movements of flexion, extension, abduction, adduction, and rotation are carried out in the foot and locomotion made possible.

Postural stability, by which is meant the maintenance of the leg in a functionally vertical position over the foot, is taken care of entirely by the long muscles. It is through postural stability that the line of transmitted weight is maintained in its proper relation to the foot when shifts in the center of gravity of the body occur as the result of changes in position.

In addition to these other functions, certain of the long muscles act as important supports in maintaining the stability of the longi-tudinal arch of the foot. The most important of the long muscles which provide support to the longitudinal arches are the tibialis anticus, the tibialis posticus, the flexor longus hallucis, the flexor longus digitorum, and the peroneus longus and tertius (Fig. 21).

The tibialis anticus, through its insertion into the internal cuneiform and first metatarsal bone, aids in supporting the inner aspect of the foot, and through this support acts in maintaining the stability of the inner longitudinal arch (Fig. 19).

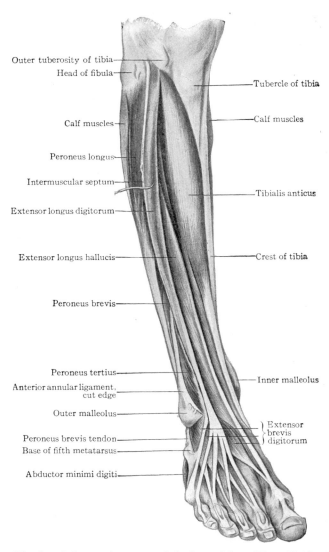

Outer tuberosity of tibia

Head of fibula

Tubercle of tibia

Calf muscles

Calf muscles

Peroneus longus

Intermuscular septum

Tibialis anticus

Extensor longus digitorum

Extensor longus hallucis

Crest of tibia

Peroneus brevis

Peroneus tertius

Inner malleolus

Anterior annular ligament, cut edge

Outer malleolus

Extensor brevis digitorum

Peroneus brevis tendon

Base of fifth metatarsus

Abductor minimi digiti

FIG. 19. Muscles of the anterior aspect of the leg and foot. (From Heisler, Practical Anatomy, J. B. Lippincott Co.)

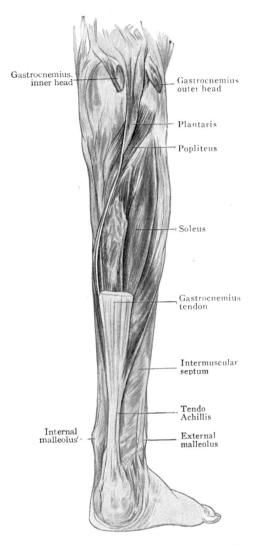

Fig. 20. Muscles and tendons on the posterior aspect of the foot and leg. (From Heisler, Practical Anatomy, J. B. Lippincott Co.)

The tibialis posticus passes under the inferior calcaneoscaphoid ligament anterior to the sustentaculum tali of the os calcis and offers strong resistance to the head of the astragalus rolling inward in weight-bearing, thus providing an important support of the inner longitudinal arch. It also supports the inner longitudinal

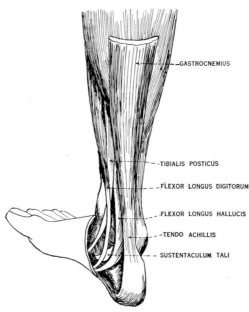

FIG. 21. Muscles on the medial and posterior aspect of the foot. (Redrawn from Davis, Applied Anatomy, J. B. Lippincott Co.)

arch through its insertion into the scaphoid and other tarsal bones (Fig. 21 and 22).

The flexor longus digitorum passes down and around the sustentaculum tali to insert into the terminal phalanges of the four outer toes. The flexor longus digitorum gives definite support to the sustentaculum tali and resists inward rotation of the os calcis and the descent of the subtalar joint; through this action it supports the longitudinal arch (Fig. 21).

The flexor longus hallucis muscle passes under the sustentaculum tali in close relation with the flexor longus digitorum and inserts into the distal phalanx of the great toe. With the foot in a passive state, this muscle acts as a flexor of the great toe and has a "grasping motion." In action such as walking or running, the

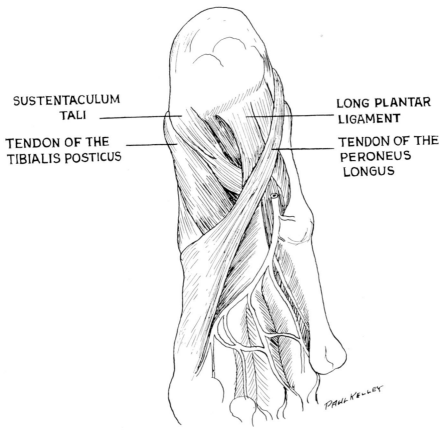

SUSTENTACULUM
TALI

TENDON OF THE
TIBIALIS POSTICUS

LONG PLANTAR
LIGAMENT

TENDON OF THE
PERONEUS
LONGUS

PAUL KELLEY

FIG. 22. Sole of the foot showing the insertion of the peroneus longus and tibialis posticus. (Redrawn after Heisler, Practical Anatomy, J. B. Lippincott Co.)

first phalanx is immobilized against the first metatarsal by the action of the short muscles of the great toe, and the flexor longus hallucis exerts a strong, propulsive action and at the same time acts as a support or elevator of the longitudinal arch by resisting inward rotation of the os calcis (Fig. 21).

Peroneus longus. The part played by the peroneus longus as a support of the arches of the foot has been debated at some length. Its course is from the outer side of the foot across the under surface of the tarsus to the inner side where it is inserted into the outer side of the base of the first metatarsal and internal cuneiform bones. From its course and sling-like position, it would seem to serve as a support to the longitudinal arch, and by its action it may possibly compress the forepart of the foot and tend to maintain the stability of the metatarsal arch (Fig. 22).

The peroneus tertius passes down in front of the external malleolus and inserts into the upper surface of the fifth metatarsal. It may tend to some extent to lift the arch upward.

It will be noted that the tendon of the tibialis anticus and peroneus tertius are practically inserted into the convexity of the longitudinal arch and tend to support it by pulling it upward. The flexor longus digitorum and flexor longus hallucis run longitudinally beneath the long arch and so directly support it. The tibialis posticus and peroneus longus from the medial and from the lateral sides respectively meet and cross on the sole of the foot and form a sling beneath the longitudinal arch (Fig. 22).

SHORT MUSCLES

The short or intrinsic muscles of the foot act very much as do the intrinsic muscles of the hand; that is, they intensify or alter the action of the long muscles, particularly in respect to the action of the long flexors and extensors on the phalanges. In addition, the intrinsic muscles of the foot act upon the metatarsal bones in such a way as to cause them to move apart or separate and relax the forepart of the foot; or they draw the metatarsals together into a firm, compact arrangement. From the manner in which these muscles act upon the metatarsal bones, it is evident that they play an important role in enabling the forepart of the foot to adapt itself to the demands of a constantly changing center of gravity and provide a definite support to the metatarsal arch by holding the heads of the metatarsal bones in firm contact when subjected to the stress of weight-bearing (Fig. 23).

BLOOD SUPPLY OF THE FOOT

The blood supply of the foot is through the anterior and posterior tibial arteries, the principal terminal branches being the

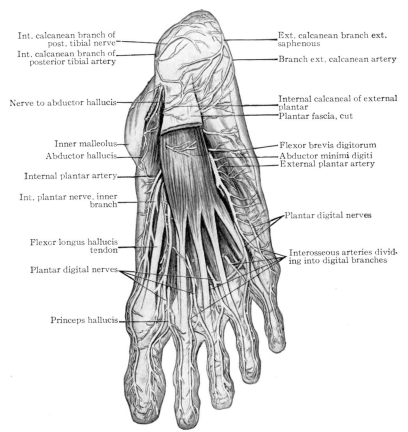

Int. calcanean branch of
    post. tibial nerve

Int. calcanean branch of
    posterior tibial artery

Nerve to abductor hallucis

Inner malleolus

Abductor hallucis

Internal plantar artery

Int. plantar nerve, inner
    branch

Flexor longus hallucis
    tendon

Plantar digital nerves

Princeps hallucis

Ext. calcanean branch ext.
saphenous

Branch ext. calcanean artery

Internal calcaneal of external
plantar

Plantar fascia, cut

Flexor brevis digitorum

Abductor minimi digiti

External plantar artery

Plantar digital nerves

Interosseous arteries dividing into digital branches

Fig. 23. Muscles of the foot, plantar view. (From Heisler, Practical Anatomy, J. B. Lippincott Co.)

dorsal pedis and the external plantar which anastomose to form several superficial and deep plantar arterial arches. The dorsalis pedis artery passes forward from the ankle along the dorsum of the foot to the base of the first intermetatarsal space. The palpation of this artery is simple, and the presence or absence of pulsation in it is frequently used as an indication as to whether the blood supply to the foot is interfered with. The plantar surface of the foot is devoid of superficial veins, but the dorsum is well drained by a venous arch, which in turn reaches the external and internal saphenous veins. The deep veins follow the course of the arteries.

NERVES OF THE FOOT

The cutaneous nerve supply of the foot is derived from terminal branches of the external and internal popliteal and the anterior crural nerves. The musculocutaneous nerve, a terminal branch of the external popliteal, supplies the major portion of the dorsum of the foot and the dorsal aspect of the second, third, fourth and the inner side of the fifth toes with their interspaces. The outer side of the fifth toe and foot are supplied by the small or external saphenous, a terminal branch of the internal popliteal. The great toe and the medial side of the second toe are supplied by a terminal branch of the anterior tibial. The medial aspect of the foot is supplied by the internal saphenous, a terminal branch of the anterior crural. The sole of the foot is supplied by terminal branches of the posterior tibial.

The muscles of the foot and lower leg receive their nerve supply from the muscular branches of the internal and external popliteal nerves.

3

PHYSIOLOGY

An understanding of the normal physiology of the ʟoot is just as necessary to an appreciation of functional disorders of the foot as a knowledge of normal anatomy is to an understanding of departures from normal in foot structure. The physiology of the foot is in reality very complex since it is called upon to function with the individual at rest and in motion. Furthermore the foot, both with the body at rest and in locomotion, is but a part of a very complex mechanism which maintains the balance of the body under constantly changing relationships between it and the external world; these are necessary to normal existence. It will be appreciated then that incoming sensory impulses, co-ordinating centers in the central nervous system, and co-ordinated motor impulses all play a part in foot function. Interesting as it might be to study these extrinsic factors concerned in foot function, it seems best to confine our discussion to the physiology of the foot alone, since a detailed study of balance and gait is so complex a subject that it had best be studied from special articles devoted to it. Plato Schwartz, Dudley Morton, Lube, and others have written extensively on this subject and their writings may be read with profit by those interested in this phase of foot physiology.

FUNCTIONS

Broadly speaking, the functions of the human foot are:

1. To provide support for the weight of the body.
2. To provide a lever to raise the body and to propel it into motion (as walking, running, jumping).
3. To act as a shock absorber for the body when it is in motion and exposed to sudden or unexpected impacts.

SUPPORTING FUNCTION

The foot fulfills its function of a support for the body both with the individual at rest and in motion. When the foot acts in this capacity, the body weight is transmitted through the ankle joint to the astragalus from which it is distributed through the arches of the foot to the three-point contact already mentioned—the os calcis, the head of the first, and the head of the fifth metatarsal bones. The three-point contact of both feet forms the base of support upon which the body rests when standing in a state of equilibrium. Because, as bipeds, we possess a sense of equilibrium, the body is held poised on its base of support and little muscular effort is necessary; in fact, just sufficient to keep the leg balanced on the astragalus. In standing, then, muscles play but little part in supporting the arches of the foot; almost the entire burden is borne by the bones and ligaments. Ligaments serve the purpose of binding bones together and preventing wide separation of bones, coupled to form joints; they are constructed to meet sudden or momentary strains, not to withstand prolonged stress.

It naturally follows then that when the foot acts as a passive support, as in standing, the ligaments are called upon to bear a strain for which they are but poorly adapted and may, if standing is too greatly prolonged, stretch and permit abnormal separation of the foot bones and induce a true foot strain. It is for this reason that foot complaints are more common among those whose occupations require long periods of standing with little opportunity for change of position, such as motormen, salespeople, etc. It is desirable, therefore, when the foot acts as a passive support, that strain on the ligaments be reduced to a minimum. Ligaments are under the least strain when the bones of the foot are so aligned that each fits into its proper place in the architectural plan, so that as the superimposed weight of the body falls upon the foot, the bones gravitate into a compact mass which is rigid and relatively non-yielding. Such a compact arrangement of the bones of the foot requires only that support from the ligaments that is necessary to hold them in their proper relationship with each other. The standing position in which the foot points straight forward or in moderate out-toeing is the position in which this locking of the bones of the foot is at its maximum and the ligaments are under the least strain (Fig. 24). With the foot in a position of eversion, i.e., with the foot turned outward, the bones instead of lying in close contact are separated, the foot is less compact, and there is a maximum of strain thrown upon the ligaments (Fig. 25). With the body at rest, the efficiency of the foot is in the main dependent upon its structural stability, that is, the integrity of the ligaments and the correct architectural arrangement of its bones.

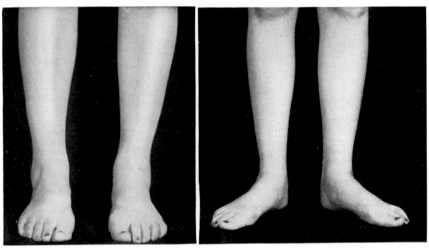

FIG. 24   FIG. 25

FIG. 24. Correct position of the feet in standing, with toes pointing forward.
FIG. 25. Incorrect position of the feet in standing, with toes pointing outward.

With the body in motion the supporting function of the foot is complicated by the fact that the body's center of gravity is constantly being displaced, and the body is continually out of equilibrium with relation to the foot. The foot under such conditions remains as a fixed base of support, but in order that the body weight may be properly distributed to it, the leg must be maintained in a functionally vertical position over it. With the body in motion, this balancing of the leg on the foot is accomplished by the tonicity of the long muscles of the foot which cross the ankle joint and stabilize the subastragalar joint—the joint through which the leg maintains its balanced position over the foot (Fig. 26).

Morton refers to this balancing of the leg on the foot as a "postural stability," a clearly descriptive term. With the body in motion, the muscles play a more important role in supporting the foot than they do with the body at rest, because of this element of postural stability. Moreover, with the body in motion, the long muscles become more important as supports of the arches, since by maintaining the leg in balance over the foot, they prevent ab-

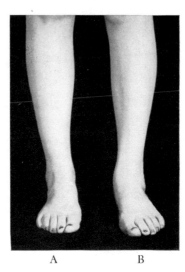

A   B

FIG. 26. A, foot in correct balance at the subastragalar joint; B, inrolling or pronation with foot out of balance at the subastragalar joint.

normal concentration of weight stresses on one part of the foot and favor their equitable distribution, thus preventing strain on the foot arches. It also seems unquestionable that with the body in motion, the muscles play a definite role in maintaining the structural stability of the foot by reason of the support which they give directly to its arches. Certainly, as we have seen in the chapter on anatomy, the course of the tendons and the action of a number of the long muscles of the foot indicate that they have very definite supporting function.

It may be said, then, that the supporting function of the foot is dependent upon both structural and postural stability. In other words, upon the proper alignment of the foot bones, integrity of the supporting ligaments, and tonicity of the leg and foot muscles.

LEVERAGE FUNCTION

When the foot acts as a lever to raise or propel the body, its role changes from a passive one, such as it fills in standing, to a kinetic one and the muscles assume major importance. In action the muscles not only provide the power which carries out the movements of the foot necessary to perform a given act but also support the arches of the foot during the carrying out of such movements. The support which is supplied to the arches of the foot by the muscles is not of the passive type to be expected from the ligaments but is an active, changing support which adapts itself to the changing relations of the bones of the foot as they move on each other in action. With the foot in action, then, the muscles are of paramount importance and a brief consideration of the movements of the foot and the most important muscles concerned in these movements is worthwhile.

MOVEMENTS

The principal movements of the foot are dorsal flexion, plantar flexion, abduction, and adduction. However, by calling into use various muscle groups and a series of joints at the same time, a wider variation of movement takes place, as metatarsal abduction, metatarsal adduction, flexion and extension of the toes, as well as a rotation of the foot in its entirety.

True plantar flexion and dorsal flexion are carried out at the ankle joint. The plantar flexors are the gastrocnemius and soleus muscles, acting through the heel tendon, and to some extent the peroneus longus and brevis muscles, and the tibialis posticus. The chief dorsal flexors of the ankle are the tibialis anticus, peroneus tertius, and the extensor communis digitorum muscles. The normal range of ankle motion is about five degrees to ten degrees past a right angle for dorsal flexion and about one hundred thirty to one hundred forty degrees of plantar flexion (Fig. 27). The range of plantar and dorsal flexion varies in the two sexes. There is a greater range of dorsal flexion in men than in women; and conversely, a greater range of plantar flexion in women than in men. When the foot is held at a right angle to the leg there is very little lateral motion in the ankle joint, this movement being prevented by the wedging of the astragalus into the ankle mortice formed by the internal and external malleoli. When the foot is

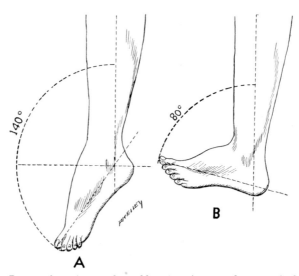

Fɪɢ. 27. Range of motion at the ankle joint. A, normal range of plantar flexion; B, normal range of dorsal flexion.

held in extreme plantar flexion, the range of lateral motion is increased owing to the narrow posterior part of the astragalus coming to lie in the ankle mortice, thus allowing more play in the ankle joint. For this reason, the ankle joint with its adjacent structures is more easily turned or sprained when the foot is in a position of plantar flexion.

True adduction and abduction or lateral movements of the foot are carried out at the subastragalar joint with the aid of the long lateral muscles (Fig. 28). As has already been stated, the leg is maintained in a balanced position over the foot by the tonicity of the leg muscles acting through the subastragalar joint. This joint then is of paramount importance in foot balance. The tibialis posticus muscle is the chief adductor or invertor and the peroneus longus and brevis muscles the main abductors or evertors. There is very little flexion and extension in this joint, the anterior and posterior calcaneo-astragaloid ligaments holding this action in check.

Movement at the midtarsal joint (astragaloscaphoid, calcaneo-

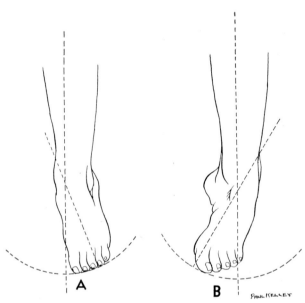

Fig. 28. Range of lateral movements of the foot. A, range of abduction; B, range of adduction.

cuboid and scaphocuneiform joints) is not a true lateral motion of abduction and adduction but rather a lateral rotating movement (Fig. 29). As the foreportion of the foot is adducted by the action of the tibialis posticus and anticus, there is also an inward rotation of this portion of the foot; and inversely, when the forefoot is abducted or everted by the action of the peroneus tertius there is an outward rotation of the forefoot.

The action of flexion and extension of the toes is carried out by the flexor longus hallucis and flexor longus digitorum and the extensor longus hallucis and the extensor longus digitorum muscles respectively. The actions of these muscles are intensified and modified by the short muscles of the foot. The flexor longus hallucis in addition to its function as a flexor of the great toe, plays an important part in walking; it forcibly flexes the great toe on the foot, in which position it is immobilized by the short muscles; continuing its action, it exerts a strong propulsive force to move the body weight forward.

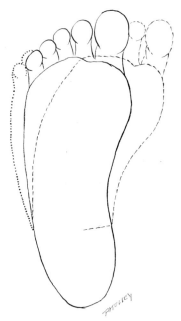

Fig. 29. Range of movement at the midtarsal joint.

Walking, Running, Etc.

Having briefly considered the major movements of the foot, we may now study these movements as they enter into the acts of walking, running, etc. Normally, as a step is taken, the heel is raised from the ground by the action of the calf muscles and the body weight rests upon the ball of the foot and toes. This action occurs in the sagittal plane until complete flexion has been accomplished, then a slight inward rotation of the foot takes place owing to the adduction action of the tibialis posticus muscle; at the same time the long and transverse arches of the foot increase in convexity. At this point, through the combined action of the heel tendon, the peroneus longus and brevis, the tibialis posticus and flexor muscles of the toes, the body weight is propelled forward. At the same time, the dorsal flexors are called into action to lift the foot so that it may clear the ground as it is swung forward to complete the step. As the heel strikes the ground, the four outer toes are flexed at the mid-phalangeal joint and extended at the distal joint, and the great toe is held in extension ready for the act of propulsion as soon as the forepart of the foot again comes in contact with the ground; as this occurs, the four outer

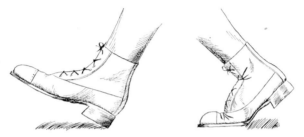

FIG. 30. Position of feet in heel-to-toe walking.

toes flex to aid the great toe in propelling the foot and body forward. This method of walking is called heel-to-toe walking, because the heel of the advancing foot first strikes the ground, and, as the body weight is thrown more and more onto the foot, it is next borne by the entire foot through the three-point contact of the sole and finally by the forepart of the foot and toes as complete plantar flexion is carried out.

Heel-to-toe walking is the form generally used in locomotion (Fig. 30). To be efficient, the foot should point directly forward in the sagittal plane with each step as shown in Fig. 31A, or at least toe out only twenty to thirty degrees. This alignment of the foot is desirable because in this position the bones of the foot are in their most favorable position mechanically, as has already been mentioned when discussing the static foot. If the foot is adducted or "toes in," the convexity of the various arches is accentuated and the foot is in a strained and cramped position (Fig. 31B). It is true that this adducted position is, from a structural point of view, a stronger position than that in which the foot is in the neutral or straight position, but the loss of flexibility and

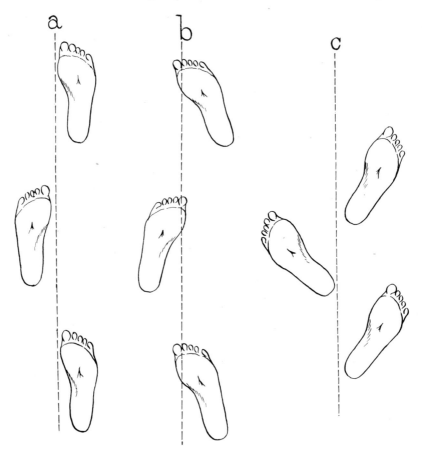

Fig. 31. Position of feet in walking. A, normal position of foot in walking with toes pointing directly forward; B, abnormal position of foot in walking with toes pointed in; C, abnormal position of foot in walking with toes pointed out.

interference with smooth action which results necessitates more work for the long and short muscles, and tends to cause foot tire and leg ache. When the foot is abducted or everted in walking (Fig. 31C), it is in the weak position since this attitude tends to separate from each other the bones which compose the arches and interferes with the compact arrangement of the foot bones so necessary to structural stability. Because the everted position results in distorting stresses upon the foot bones, it places an excessive strain on the ligaments of the foot which bind these bones together. If such abnormal strain on the ligaments is maintained constantly over long periods of time, the ligaments stretch and elongate and their efficiency is lessened; this in turn calls for an excessive amount of effort on the part of the muscles of the foot to compensate for the inefficiency of the ligaments. Constantly walking with the foot everted leads to ligamentous strain, muscle

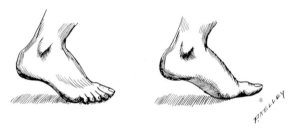

FIG. 32. Position of foot in toe-to-toe walking.

tire, and may eventually cause impairment of the entire architecture of the foot.

When all of the weight is borne on the ball of the foot as in walking on "tip toe," it is called toe-to-toe walking (Fig. 32). Toe-to-toe walking imparts greater elasticity and spring to the gait and results in less shock impact than heel-to-toe walking because with the weight borne entirely on the ball of the foot, almost the entire burden of weight-bearing is thrown upon the muscles, the metatarsal heads alone of the bones of the foot taking any part in carrying the body weight. Because of the added elasticity and spring which is secured by toe-to-toe walking, it is used in running, and because it is more graceful, it is used in dancing. Toe-to-toe walking is, however, more tiring than heel-to-toe walking because of the increased burden thrown upon the foot and leg muscles and cannot be employed for sustained and continuous locomotion.

SHOCK-ABSORBING FUNCTION

The shock-absorbing qualities of the foot lie in its structural design. The accurate articulation of the foot bones with each other makes for strength. The play or movement between the individual bones of the foot, permitted by the numerous joints, provides for flexibility and resiliency which enable the foot to absorb shocks and jars. In addition, the arrangement of the foot bones in the form of arches provides a structural device which allows greater play between the individual bones of the foot than would be possible by any other arrangement and adds to the resiliency of the foot. The arch formation also distributes stresses, strains, and shocks over the entire foot in an equable manner so that each part bears its portion and no part is called upon to bear more than its share. We have, then, in the foot an organ well adapted by reason of its architecture and construction to cushion stresses, strains, and impacts which, with a less efficient form of construction, would be transmitted to the legs, torso, and head in all their intensity. The foot with its arches may be compared to the springs of a motor car in that it absorbs shocks and jars incident to locomotion and general activity. Anyone who has ridden in a vehicle which is without springs can readily appreciate how important they are in saving wear and tear and in preventing actual discomfort; we would be in almost the same plight without the shock-absorbing qualities of the foot.

SUMMARY

The functions of the human foot are support, leverage, and shock absorption, and these functions are necessary for comfortable and efficient living. In order that each of these functions may be properly performed, a normal arrangement of the intrinsic osteo-articular structure of the foot must be present combined with a properly balanced extrinsic musculotendinous structure. With such a combination, the foot and leg are in balance, body weight is distributed evenly over the foot and it functions with ease and efficiency as an organ of support, as a propulsive lever, and as a shock absorber. It is equally true that either a faulty osteo-articular or musculotendinous arrangement or a combination of these will interfere with normal action of the foot and bring about a perverted or abnormal physiology. Factors which may bring about disturbance in the normal physiology of the foot will be considered in the chapter on "Primary Causes of Foot Imbalance," page 46.

4

PRIMARY CAUSES OF FOOT IMBALANCE

The anatomy and physiology of the normal foot have been discussed so far as seems necessary to an understanding of the foot as an organ of support and locomotion. The next study to engage us is that of departures from normal in its anatomy and physiology which are responsible for functional foot disorders. These disorders have been grouped together under the term "Imbalance." In the discussion of each type of foot imbalance, the specific etiologic factors responsible will be gone into in detail. It seems desirable, however, before taking up the discussion of the various functional foot disorders to discuss certain structural defects of the foot which cause disturbance in its normal mechanism and may, therefore, be looked upon as primary causal factors in the production of foot imbalance. These primary causative factors, if not entirely responsible for symptomatic foot disorders, at least play a very important role, and the manner in which they affect foot balance should be thoroughly understood.

The ability of the foot to function effectively as a base of support, as a lever to propel the body, and as a shock absorber depends, as so ably pointed out by Morton, upon two elements: structural stability and postural stability. By structural stability is meant the quality which enables it to provide a rigid base of support in all directions for the superimposed body weight. By postural stability is meant that quality whereby the center of transmitted weight is constantly maintained in a balanced position over the astragalus with each shift of the body's center of gravity.

STRUCTURAL STABILITY

Structural stability is supplied by the bones and the ligaments which bind these bones together. This is not entirely true because even with the body at rest a certain amount of muscle effort is necessary to maintain the leg in balance over the foot. As structural stability is mainly dependent upon the integrity of the bones and ligaments of the foot, it follows that any abnormality in the form of the bones of the foot will result in a defective architecture and a lessening of structural stability. It is equally true that any weakness or loss of tone in the ligaments of the foot will result in a lessening of the strength and effectiveness of these important supports of the arches, will allow abnormal separation between the bones, and will contribute to the loss of structural stability. Loss of structural stability results in faulty foot balance.

POSTURAL STABILITY

Postural stability is maintained through the action of the short intrinsic muscles of the foot, and more particularly through the tonicity of the long muscles of the leg and foot which pass across the ankle joint. It is through the tonicity of these muscles that the leg is maintained in a functionally vertical position over the foot with each shift of the body weight. Any weakness or loss of balance in the foot and leg muscle groups will disturb the normal balance of the leg on the foot and cause a breakdown of postural stability. Loss of postural stability results in unequal distribution of weight stresses over the foot and tends to weaken structural stability.

FACTORS IN STABILITY

From the foregoing comments it is evident that: (1) Any factor which decreases structural stability will make postural stability more difficult to maintain and will increase the work required of the foot and leg muscles. (2) Any disturbance of postural stability will result in an unequal distribution of weight stresses over the foot, put an unusual strain upon the ligaments which may eventually stretch and relax and bring about a breakdown in structural stability. Broadly viewed, then, it may be stated that any condition which interferes sufficiently with either structural or postural stability of the foot is a cause of foot imbalance. More specifically stated, defective architecture owing to abnormalities involving the bones of the foot, relaxation or loss of elasticity of the ligaments and paralysis, weakness, or loss of balance between antagonistic muscle groups of the foot or leg are the primary causes of foot imbalance and lead to functional foot disorders.

DEFECTS IN BONY ARCHITECTURE

Occasionally, distortions of one or more bones of the foot occur as developmental defects; such distortions may result in serious interference with foot architecture and cause faulty foot balance. There are four weaknesses in the bony structure of the foot which lessen structural stability. These are: (1) Shortness of the first metatarsal bone; (2) hypermobility of the first metatarsal bone or segment; (3) metatarsus varus primus; and (4) accessory scaphoid or prehallux. To Dudley Morton must go the credit for emphasizing the importance of the first two of these conditions. Lapidus has emphasized the importance of the third condition. Kidner, Haglund, Froelich, and others have discussed the fourth.

Shortness of the first metatarsal bone, a developmental condition, is found in a certain per cent of unbalanced feet, possibly 50 per cent or more (Fig. 33). This shortness may be as great as one centimeter. When the first metatarsal bone is short, it fails to come properly into contact with the bearing surface and sustain its share of the superimposed weight; this results in a concentration of weight stresses on the relatively long second metatarsal bone, which hypertrophies and becomes more robust (Fig. 33). Also, when the first metatarsal bone is short, the foot must roll inward in order that the head of the bone may come in contact with the weight-bearing surface; this brings about a greater or lesser degree of pronation of the foot, depending upon the amount of shortness of the first metatarsal present. Shortness of the first metatarsal bone and hypertrophy of the second metatarsal can be clearly demonstrated, when present, by a dorsoplantar x-ray of the foot taken in weight-bearing. It is quite evident that such a definite structural defect must be a very important primary cause of foot imbalance, since it favors inrolling of the foot, unequal and abnormal weight distribution over the foot, and ligamentous strain.

Dorsal hypermobility of the first metatarsal segment (first metatarsal with its digit and the medial cuneiform bone) due to an unusual amount of mobility in the joints between the scaphoid and the medial and middle cuneiform bone, produces about the same effect as does a short first metatarsal in that the first metatarsal fails to carry its proper proportion of the superimposed weight. This avoidance of weight-bearing by the first metatarsal head is made possible by the following: When the heads of the

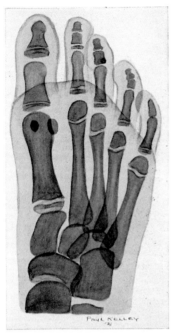

FIG. 33. Tracing of dorsiplantar x-ray of foot showing shortness of the first metatarsal bone.

other metatarsals, which are not relaxed, come in contact with the bearing surface, the first metatarsal simply continues to flex dorsally by reason of its abnormal mobility. The head then becomes ineffective as a weight-bearing point because the normal degree of stability usually supplied by the first metatarsal segment is lacking. When such a condition exists, the anterior pier of the internal longitudinal arch (head of the first metatarsal bone) is lacking in stability, the foot rolls inward or pronates, and excessive stress is thrown upon the ligaments and muscles. Laxness of the first metatarsal segment is indicated when a dorsi-plantar x-ray of the foot, taken in weight-bearing, shows an un-usual degree of separation between the medial and middle cuneiform bones (Fig. 34).

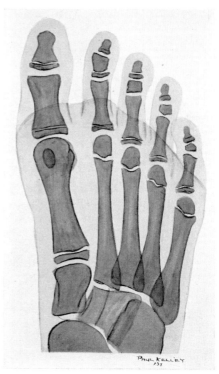

FIG. 34. Tracing of a dorsiplantar x-ray of a foot showing a separation between the medial and middle cuneiform bones which denotes a laxness of the first metatarsal segment.

Metatarsus varus primus is a developmental condition which is a throwback to the arboreal foot. With metatarsus varus primus, the first metatarsal bone projects medially at a more acute angle than normal, the projection inward starting at the joint between the first metatarsal and medial cuneiform bone (Fig. 35). Owing to the increased angularity of the first metatarsal bone, there is a wide interspace between the first and second metatarsal bones and the forepart of the foot is broadened or splayed out. Almost invariably metatarsus varus primus deformity is associated with laxness or hypermobility in the first metatarsal segment. The resemblance between a foot in which metatarsus varus primus is present, and the arboreal foot with its divergent and extremely mobile first metatarsal is at once evident. The authors have observed a family of three children who showed gradations of metatarsus varus primus from

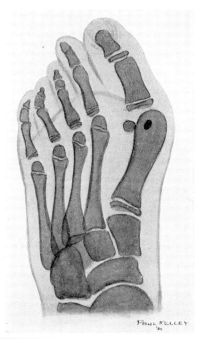

FIG. 35. Tracing of a dorsiplantar x-ray taken in weight-bearing, showing the medial deviation of the first metatarsal bone—metatarsus varus primus.

a moderate degree of deformity in the oldest child to a true grasping arboreal foot in the youngest child; in fact, the youngest child was said to have strangled a puppy by squeezing its neck between the first and second toes. Such a combination of increased angularity of the first metatarsal bone and increased mobility of the first metatarsal segment interferes with the mechanics of the foot in two ways. Increased medial angulation of the first metatarsal bone broadens out the forepart of the foot and leaves a wide interspace between the digits of the first and second meta-

tarsal bones and when a shoe is worn the mobile great toe, im-
pelled by the pressure of the side of the shoe and disturbed muscle
pull, tends to migrate laterally to fill up this space, and hallux
valgus deformity or bunion results. Lateral migration of the digit
of the first metatarsal deprives the inner longitudinal arch of a
definitely stabilizing support and favors pronation. The hypermobility of the first metatarsal segment which is associated with
metatarsus varus primus interferes with the mechanics of the foot
in the same way as does a hypermobile first metatarsal segment
uncomplicated by a metatarsus varus primus, in that the head of
the first metatarsal bone does not properly contact the bearing
surface due to its lack of rigidity and the anterior pier of the inner
longitudinal arch (the head of the first metatarsal bone) is unstable. With instability of the anterior pier of the inner longitudinal arch, the foot rolls downward and inward or pronates
under the stress of weight-bearing and there is excessive strain on
the ligaments and muscles.

Accessory scaphoid, or prehallux, is an architectural defect
which interferes with the structural stability in the foot. The
prehallux is a supernumerary bone which appears occasionally in
the human foot, attached to or fused with the inner border of
the scaphoid (Fig. 36). When a prehallux is present, the tendon
of the tibialis posticus on its way to its final insertion into the
internal cuneiform and first metatarsal, attaches to it instead of to
the under surface of the scaphoid tubercle. Kidner states that because of the abnormal attachment of the tendon of the tibialis
posticus, the line of pull is changed so that instead of pulling
directly upward as it normally does, it pulls backward and inward
at an angle and becomes a pronator instead of a supinator. This,
of course, makes it work at a mechanical disadvantage, and it
must work harder to accomplish an equal lift on the tarsus.
Second, the long lever arm of the prehallux turning inward forces
the muscle to greater lineal contraction in order to produce a
given amount of lift at the center of the arch. In other words, the
lifting effect on the arch is reduced first by the angulation of the
line of pull, and second, by the longer distance through which the
pull must act. Third, the effort to lift the arch or adduct the foot

is very quickly stopped by the close approach of the prehallux to the internal malleolus. Fourth, the crowding of the tissues between the prehallux and internal malleolus causes discomfort which is automatically relieved by abduction or pronation of the foot. It will be seen then that prehallux has definite possibilities as a causative factor in the production of foot imbalance.

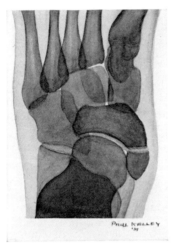

FIG. 36. Tracing of a dorsiplantar x-ray showing an accessory scaphoid or prehallux.

RELAXATION OF LIGAMENTS

Relaxation of the ligaments of the foot may be a part of a general relaxation, a condition which is by no means rare in the slender, small-boned type of individual. Ligamentous relaxation may also be the result of undue strain put upon the foot by an excessive increase in body weight; it may result from arthritic or toxic conditions; it may follow overworking the foot in certain types of occupation, notably those which require long periods of standing or use of the foot under abnormal conditions.

Relaxation of important supporting ligaments permits separation of the bones of the foot to a degree which prevents them from maintaining the firm, compact arrangement which is necessary for structural stability. Loss of structural stability means eventually loss of or interference with postural stability and foot strain (Fig. 37). If ligaments lose their normal elasticity, they prevent normal movement between the bones of the foot, lessen its flexibility and adaptability, and so interfere with both structural and postural stability and foot strain results.

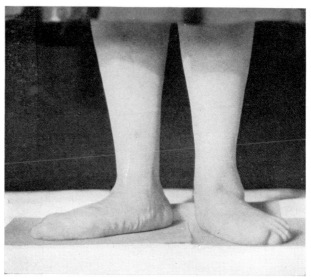

Fig. 37. Extreme relaxation of the foot; flaccid flatfoot.

MUSCLE IMBALANCE

Paralysis of muscles or muscle groups results from infantile paralysis, nerve injuries, or diseases of the central nervous system. Weakness of muscle groups may result from debilitating diseases or from long periods of inactivity. Paralysis or weakness of muscle groups interferes with or prevents balance of the leg over the foot and so results in a serious disturbance of postural stability, which in turn leads to abnormal weight distribution over the foot with eventual breaking down of structural stability and foot strain. Loss of balance between antagonistic muscle groups occurs in spastic paralysis but is seen in its most common form when a congenitally short heel cord or overdeveloped calf muscle interferes with the normal anterior-posterior balance of the foot. A short heel cord or overactive calf muscle disturbs balance by lifting the heel from the ground, thus reducing the arc of dorsal flexion, and putting abnormal strain upon the foot structures, particularly the forefoot. In both standing and walking, lessening of the dorsal flexion of the foot results in a powerful leverage strain on the astragalus (talus) which tends to roll downward and inward and produce strain on the structures forming the longitudinal arch.

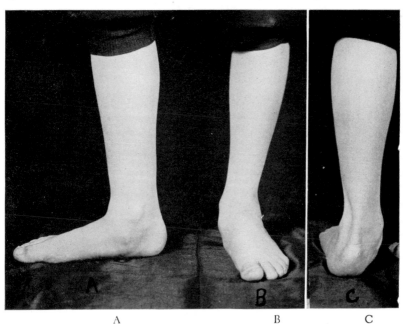

A   B   C

Fig. 38. Flaccid flatfoot; result of muscle imbalance. A, depression of the longitudinal arch; B, inrolling of the foot or pronation; C, tensity and lateral deviation of the heel cord.

If such an abnormal strain continues over a sufficiently long period of time, weakening and depression of the longitudinal arch will result (Fig. 38). Muscle imbalance, then, from whatever cause, interferes with or destroys postural and eventually structural stability and tends to bring about a breakdown of the entire foot structure.

SUMMARY

Architectural defects involving the bony structures of the foot, ligamentous weakness or loss of elasticity, and muscle imbalance are the primary causative factors underlying most functional foot disorders. All can bring about faulty distribution of weight stresses over the foot, which, if sufficiently long continued, interferes with the normal mechanics of the foot and leads eventually to disabling foot disorders. It is probable that structural defects alone are not sufficient to produce symptomatic foot disorders in most cases but merely "set the stage" in that a potentially weak foot results from the faulty mechanics for which they are responsible. When, however, such a potentially weak foot is called upon to function in faulty footwear, through long hours of labor, and under unfavorable environmental conditions, or is further weakened by debilitating constitutional conditions, it is to be expected that it will prove unequal to the demands made upon it and give way and become symptom producing.

EXAMINATION

As is true in making any medical examination, a carefully taken history should precede the inspection of the feet in functional foot disorders. Such a history should include important facts in the family and past medical history of the patient and an accurate and detailed investigation of the complaints for which advice is sought.

HISTORY

The family history may give important leads pointing toward inherited conditions and family characteristics. While perhaps less important than in general medical conditions, past history is worthy of careful investigation. It is useful in that it should give information concerning the patient's general condition, reveal the presence of pre-existing disease, such as arthritis, which may have a definite bearing upon the symptoms complained of and should give important general information of service in evaluating the condition of the foot. A careful inquiry into the condition of the throat, nose, and teeth should be included in taking the past medical history; these regions are frequently the site of focal infection, and focal infection may be an important contributing factor in functional foot disorders.

The history of the present illness or complaint should be taken with care and in detail. The duration of the condition should be clearly established and whether it has been stationary or progressive in character. The area of chief discomfort and associated areas of minor discomfort, such as pain in the calf of the leg, knees, and back, should be definitely localized. The character of the pain, whether constant or intermittent, and whether aggravated or not by activity should be carefully recorded. In short, a searching inquiry should be made not only into the local complaints but into all possible associated disorders and carefully noted in the history of the present illness. The importance of a reasonably complete history can not be overemphasized, since a carelessly taken and inadequate history overlooks facts which have a definite bearing on the condition under investigation.

If the history suggests that the general health of the individual may have some connection with the foot disorder complained of, a general physical examination should be made, and be sufficiently exhaustive definitely to give the necessary information. It is also advisable to make an examination of the mouth and throat for possible foci of infection even if the patient declares that he has had no trouble with the throat or nose, nor has he any devitalized teeth. Frequently conditions are found which require attention.

It seems worthwhile here to emphasize the truism that to approach the examination of a foot which is the site of a functional disorder from the point of view of its mechanics alone, is but half to do the job. The fact that the foot is but a part of the whole and suffers along with other regions of the body from the effects of constitutional disorders can not be overlooked; failure to realize this fact in planning the treatment of any foot disability is to court failure more often than is generally appreciated, to the detriment of the patient and the reputation of the medical attendant.

EXAMINATION

When the history has been taken and when such general examinations as seem necessary have been completed, the examination of the foot may be proceeded with. This examination can be made with the patient standing on the floor in front of the examiner, but it can be made much more efficiently and comfortably by using an examining stand or platform. A stand which we have found useful can be made quite cheaply and adds greatly to the ease and efficiency of examination.

The examining stand shown in Fig. 39 has the following construction. The platform is three feet square and twenty inches high. Upon the platform is placed a chair which may be fixed or movable. Placed beneath the platform is a roll of ordinary white wrapping paper, which is threaded through a slot in the platform at about its center and passes forward to be caught in a slot at the front of the platform. This paper provides a clean white surface upon which diagrams or pedographs can be made; this may be torn off and recorded with the history if desired. A roll of adhesive

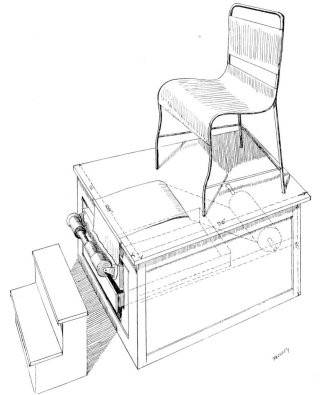

FIG. 39. Foot-examining stand. (See text for description.)

is held on a rack fixed on the front face of the stand, and a drawer just beneath this rack contains small instruments, scissors, measuring rules, and tapes. A combination step and seat allows the patient to mount the examining stand and also serves the examiner as a seat.

The patient to be examined is asked to remove both shoes and hose and to stand facing the examiner with toes pointing forward, the feet parallel, and about four inches apart. The skirt or trousers should be so arranged as to expose the feet and legs beyond the knees (Fig. 40).

A systematic method of examination should be determined upon and routinely carried out. By following a routine the ground will be completely covered, and there is less possibility of over-

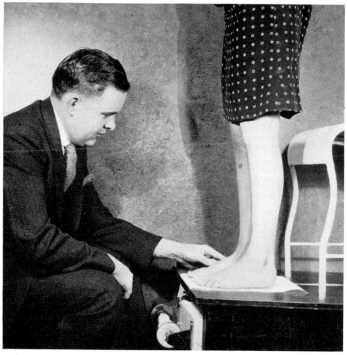

FIG. 40. Position of the examiner and patient in making an examination of the feet

looking conditions which may have a very definite relation to the cause of the trouble for which the patient is seeking advice. We have found the following form of examination satisfactory:

1. **General inspection of the feet and legs.** This should include the presence of swelling, general or localized; vascular condition of the skin; the presence of knock knee, bow leg, or torsion of the tibia; the presence of hallux valgus, corns, callosities and hammertoes, and the weight-bearing relation of the foot to the leg. If knock

knee is present, the distance between the internal malleoli should be measured with the internal condyles of
the femora in contact. If bow leg is present, the distance
between the internal condyles, the crests of the tibiae,
and the internal malleoli should be taken with the feet
placed side by side and in close contact. Such measurements constitute a record of abnormalities present
which affect the weight-bearing line of the legs and are
useful in determining the type of treatment to be used.

2. **Examination of the stance or relation of the foot to
the line of transmitted weight through the leg.** This
should include a record of any pronation (inrolling) or
eversion (outrolling) of the foot present, and the degree; mild, moderate or severe. A notation of any adduction or eversion present in the forefoot should be made.

3. **Examination of the longitudinal arch of the foot.**
In examining the longitudinal arch, the general character of the foot should be taken into consideration,
since there is considerable variation in the height of the
longitudinal arch in different feet, i.e., what seems to be
a low arch may be a normal arch for that particular foot.
The height of the longitudinal arch should be recorded
as normal, depressed, or elevated, and the degree of the
depression or elevation indicated as mild, moderate, or
severe. Some prefer to use the terms, first, second, and
third degree in describing the depression of the longitudinal arch as a convenient method of recording the
condition present.

4. **Examination of the metatarsal or transverse arch.**
With the patient sitting, some idea of the condition of
the transverse or metatarsal arch may be gained by ob-
serving whether the bones are spread apart, indicating
relaxation, or crowded together with the toes curled
up in the hammertoe position, indicating a descent of
the arch. The presence of abnormal mobility or rigidity
between the metatarsal heads should be determined.
The height of the arch should be estimated. Normally,
when sitting, the heads of the metatarsal bones form an
arch dorsally convex; if, instead of this normal arrangement, the heads of the metatarsal bones form a plantar

convex arch and the ball of the foot is prominent and calloused, the metatarsal arch should be set down as depressed.

5. **Examination for structural defects.** Shortness of the first metatarsal bone is indicated when the great toe is definitely shorter than the second toe. Hypermobility of the first metatarsal segment is suggested when there is abnormal mobility of the first metatarsal, in that it has a greater range of dorsal flexion when forced than do the other metatarsal bones. Metatarsus varus primus alters the conformation of the forepart of the foot, which becomes broad across the ball, owing to the inward projection of the first metatarsal. There is a wide interspace between the first and second toes; and the great toe tends to displace laterally and cause the great toe joint to be prominent. Undue prominence of the scaphoid bone should arouse the suspicion of an accessory scaphoid bone or prehallux.

6. **Examination of the toes.** This should include an investigation for arthritic changes in the joints, hammertoes, corns between the toes, the common site of which is between the fourth and fifth toes, and any evidence of pressure on the tuberosity of the fifth metatarsal. If a bunion is present, the amount of exostosis, the condition of the bursa over the exostosis, the degree of lateral deviation of the great toe, and whether metatarsus varus primus is present should be recorded.

7. **Examination of the heel tendon.** In making this examination, the tension of the heel tendon should be studied. In the male foot, with the knee extended, the heel tendon should allow dorsal flexion of the inverted foot to ten degrees to fifteen degrees less than a right angle; in the female foot to five degrees to ten degrees less than a right angle. This measurement is best made with an ordinary carpenters' rule with an angle measuring attachment (Fig. 41). While the measurement is being made, the patient should be questioned as to whether holding the foot in the acute dorsally flexed position causes pulling or discomfort in the calf of the

leg; if discomfort is present, it is helpful in determining
to what extent the short heel tendon may be a factor
in the foot condition complained of. The bearing which
shortening of the heel tendon has upon foot imbalance
will be discussed later.

8. Examination of the plantar fascia. This examination
   should include a determination of the tone of the plantar
   fascia, that is, whether it is normal, relaxed, or con-

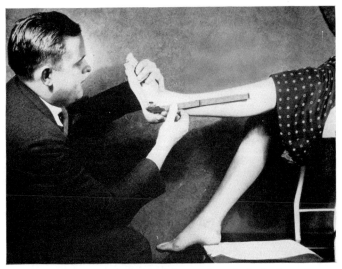

FIG. 41. Method of measuring the tension of the heel tendon.

tracted. Points of tenderness to pressure should be
sought, particularly at the insertion of the plantar fascia
into the os calcis.

9. Pedograph. A pedograph or outline of the foot in the
   weight-bearing position is not essential, but such an
   outline is a useful part of the record. The outline of the
   foot is best taken by having the patient stand on a large
   inked pad and then make an imprint of the foot on a
   suitable piece of paper which may be filed with the record (Fig. 42).

10. Examination of gait. With the shoes removed, the pa-
    tient should walk about at the ordinary gait, and the
    manner in which the foot is used should be observed.

The behavior of the foot during locomotion, i.e., whether the arch is of normal height or depressed, and the direction in which the toes point, forward or outward, often gives important information.

11. **Roentgenological examination.** A dorsoplantar x-ray of both feet in weight-bearing should always be made if possible. Such a plate will show the presence of a short

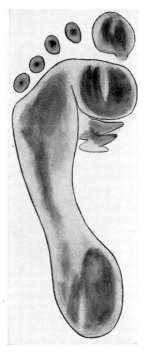

FIG. 42. Recorded pedograph of a normal foot.

first metatarsal bone, give definite information as to the distribution of weight upon the five metatarsals, and reveal looseness of the first metatarsal segment, metatarsus varus primus, and accessory scaphoid if these conditions are present. Such additional roentgenograms as may seem necessary should be taken; the conditions present will generally determine the views which will be most helpful.

12. **A study of the shoes** is well worthwhile, since the man-

ner in which the heel, sole, and uppers are worn gives valuable information regarding weight-bearing tendencies and such information may be helpful in solving the problem of foot imbalance in the foot under investigation.

6

THE FOOT OF CHILDHOOD

THE FOOT OF THE INFANT

The normal foot at birth is complete in all of its elements, but still in a plastic state ready to take the form which the stresses and strains of use may determine. It is evident then that from early life the manner in which the foot is used is important, because of the influence of use on development. Furthermore, the aphorism "As the twig bends, so does the tree incline," certainly has a direct application to the development of the foot through the years of its growth, since the child's foot is the forerunner of the adult form. Indeed, there can be little doubt in the mind of any careful student of foot imbalance that many of the faults in the adult foot which underlie functional foot disorders can be traced directly to failure to recognize and correct in childhood faulty tendencies in foot development. An understanding, then, of the general development of the foot in childhood and how development may best be guided along normal lines is important and will be dealt with in some detail.

During the first months of life, the foot is not called upon to function in its weight-bearing capacity. Movements of the foot and toes during this period, however, serve the very important purpose of developing the foot bones, exercising the foot and leg muscles, building up tone in the ligaments, and generally preparing the foot for its life work of weight-bearing and locomotion.

THE FOOT AT WALKING AGE

At the age of ten to twelve months when the child begins to walk, the bones of the foot are only partially ossified, are in reality but an orderly arrangement of cartilaginous masses (Fig. 43). Only the astragalus, os calcis, external cuneiform and cuboid of the tarsal bones show centers of ossification at this time; those for the other bones do not appear until two to three years later. The muscles of the foot and leg are not yet trained to function efficiently, and the ligaments lack the toughness and strength necessary to hold the bones of the foot firmly in contact with each other. It may be accepted then that, at the walking age, the foot is still very malleable and readily influenced by the stresses placed upon it in standing and in moving the body weight from place to place. It seems quite obvious, therefore, that from the

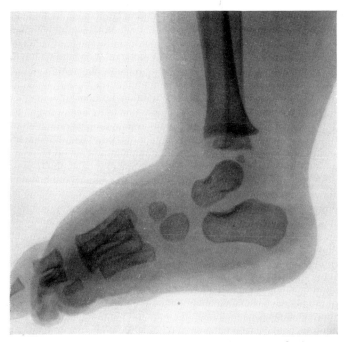

FIG. 43. X-ray of a foot at the age of one year. There are only four centers of ossification present in the tarsal bones.

beginning of weight-bearing, it is important that the foot be used in a position which insures that the stresses placed upon it will not tend to distort nor deform its still-developing structures. Stated in another way, it is important that from the beginning of weight-bearing, the foot should be used in a position of correct balance. Such a position aligns the bones of the foot in the most advantageous relationship with each other and so favors their normal growth; reduces strain on developing muscles; throws less stress on consolidating ligaments;—in brief, gives the developing foot a chance to grow into the kind of structurally strong unit it is intended to be. Failure to protect the growing foot from weakening or deforming weight stresses will result in faulty development, a weak architecture, and eventually a foot incapable of standing up under the strain of use. Prevention is always better than cure and often easier of accomplishment. Logically, then, there should be no part of the child's physical development more closely watched than that of the foot to the end that incorrect tendencies in development may be recognized early and corrective measures taken. An inquiry into what constitutes incorrect tendencies in a growing foot and the means available for their correction is, therefore, worthwhile.

LINE OF TRANSMITTED WEIGHT

When the child takes its first steps, its sense of equilibrium is rudimentary, and, uncertain in its balance, it instinctively places the feet wide apart to secure as broad a base of support as possible (Fig. 44). With the feet so separated, the line of transmitted weight falls through the great toe or medial to it, and the major part of the body weight is concentrated on the medial side of the foot which reacts in a very definite manner to the burden thus unevenly distributed to it. The primary reaction is a rolling inward and downward or pronation of the foot. Secondary to this pronation, the foot flattens out, and no longitudinal arch is evident because the ligaments, in their still undeveloped state, and the untrained leg and foot muscles are unable to withstand the excess strain put upon them and fail to hold the bones of the foot in the compact arch arrangement which weight-bearing demands. The child at this stage walks with a clumsy, flatfooted gait, and there is little spring in his step. Gradually, as the child's sense of equilibrium develops and he becomes more confident, the feet are placed closer together, and the body weight is shifted more toward the lateral side of the foot. As this shift in the body weight takes place, the line of transmitted weight approaches its proper position and falls between the first and second toes instead of falling through the great toe or medial to it. With this change in the distribution of weight stresses, the foot comes into better balance, the burden on the medial side of the foot lessens, and the pronation or the inward and downward rolling of the foot disappears. With continued use, the muscles function more

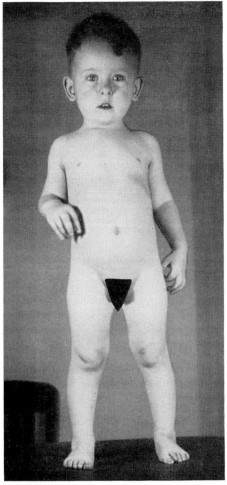

FIG. 44. As the child takes his first steps he instinctively places the feet wide apart to secure a broad base of support.

efficiently in keeping the leg balanced over the foot, the ligaments tighten, the foot becomes more compact and stronger, the superfluous fat disappears, and the arch of the foot begins to take form (Fig. 45). The child now rises on his toes with each step; there is a spring to his gait, and he walks with growing ease and confidence.

If, for any reason (and there are a number), the body weight continues to be borne preponderantly on the medial side of the foot, the inrolling or pronation persists (Fig. 46). This position of the foot, as has already been stated, tends to separate the bones of the foot and to prevent them from drawing together into a compact arrangement, places a distorting stress on the ligaments, throws an excess strain on the muscles, and interferes with the development of structural stability which is essential to an efficiently functioning foot. The foot under such conditions fails to develop normally, remains relaxed and flat and there is little or no tendency for a longitudinal arch to develop (Fig. 46). Such a foot is insufficient and incapable of functioning properly. Furthermore, if allowed to continue in this condition unchecked, an adolescent and eventually an adult flatfoot is inevitable.

The detection of undue prolongation of the early flatfooted attitude in a child's foot is possible if an examination of the foot is made a part of the routine general examination usually given at intervals. Since the pediatrician sees and examines the child during this period, the responsibility of recognizing that a foot is not developing properly must be placed upon him. Unquestionably in the past, many pediatricians have failed to give to the development of the child's foot the attention which it deserves, and there has also been failure on the part of the parents to realize its importance. In recent years, however, the picture has changed. Not only are the pediatricians looking more carefully for evidence of faulty foot balance in children, but parents, educated by publicity on foot disorders, are giving much more attention to their children's feet, and better things may therefore be looked for in the future.

Recently, several writers have taken the position that congenital flatfoot is a definite entity. There can be no doubt that congenital variations in the shape of the bones of the foot do occur. A long astragalus with a long, narrow neck, twisted externally in relation to the body, will compel an arrangement of

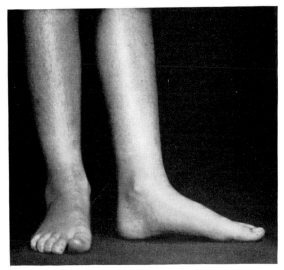

FIG. 45. Child's feet showing very little pronation and normal longitudinal arch

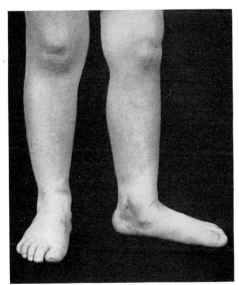

FIG. 46. Pes planus or flatfoot in the child. The longitudinal arch is depressed and there is pronation present.

the tarsal bones which will hold the tarsus permanently in valgus and the foot in pronation. Such a foot should be classified as a congenital flatfoot. Another group will show extreme and persistent relaxation of the ligaments which may be so extreme as to allow the dorsum of the foot to be brought into contact with the anterolateral surface of the tibia and complete downward displacement of the medial tarsal bones on weight-bearing. It seems questionable, however, whether this latter group should be considered to be a congenital flatfoot, since, usually, the same relaxation of ligamentous structures is found generally distributed over the entire body (Ehlers-Danlos syndrome).

The extremely relaxed type of foot in childhood should respond to those corrective measures which are advocated in the relaxed and pronating foot of childhood. A true congenital flatfoot arising from congenital variation or malformation of the astragalus or other tarsal bones should receive conservative treatment in the form of protection through the growing years, but can be expected to respond only to remodeling operations carried out later at the appropriate time.

While it is permissible to perform surgical operations on the foot of a child when such procedures are carried out on the skin, ligaments, or muscles, it is not wise to perform any operation on the bones or joints of the foot until the child has reached the age of six or better eight years. Previous to this age, the bones are largely cartilaginous and so unsatisfactory material for such surgical procedures which rely upon bony fusion for a successful result. It is, therefore, best to delay operation for the correction of congenital club foot until the child has reached the age of six years or over.

CORRECTION OF DEVELOPING FOOT FAULTS

Once it has been determined that a child's foot is not developing properly, measures should be taken to correct the faults present. This is best accomplished by prescribing a correct shoe for the child. Those of the profession who are interested in general and foot posture have given considerable thought to the type

of shoe best adapted to the growing foot, but there is still considerable difference of opinion among them as to whether a rigid
or flexible shoe is preferable. Without entering at this time into a
discussion of the advantages claimed for each type, the following
suggestions are made for the kind of shoe which should be worn
before and after the walking age.

SHOES

From birth until the walking age (ten to twelve months), the
most important requisite in foot covering is that it be loose and

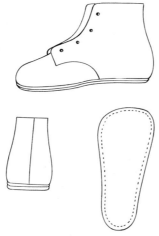

FIG. 47. A soft-sole, wide-toed shoe may be worn from birth until the walking age

flexible in order that the movements of the foot and toes be as
little restricted as possible. Exercise during this period is most
important for the development of the foot. If a shoe is worn, it
should be of a soft-sole, flexible construction, as no support is
needed (Fig. 47).

When weight-bearing starts, the environment of the foot
changes materially, and it has an entirely new set of conditions to
meet. Even under these new conditions, it must be admitted that
probably the most desirable course to follow would be to avoid
shoes and to allow the child to go barefoot so that foot develop-

ment could progress unhampered by the restricting influence of hose and shoes. This would certainly be so if the child's activities were carried out solely on springy turf or sandy beaches. Unfortunately, such conditions do not exist in modern life, as most of the child's weight-bearing is on hard and non-resilient surfaces, which, lacking give and elasticity, instead of providing a suitable medium for exercise and development, put an additional strain on the growing foot from which it must be protected by shoes. In addition, custom has decreed that children shall wear shoes. From the weight-bearing age on, then, both by custom and from necessity, the child's foot must be encased in a shoe, which, because it restricts freedom of movement and gives support, interferes to some extent with the normal development of the foot. To this extent, the foot of the modern child is weak in comparison to the foot of the barefoot races.

CRITERIA OF A CORRECT SHOE

Because of the conditions under which the child of today lives, the shoes worn by the growing child should do three things: first, they should protect the feet from traumatizing contact with hard, unyielding surfaces; second, they should provide support to make up for any insufficiency in the foot caused by restraint on development; third, they should hold the feet in a position of balance so that they may be relieved of distorting stresses and develop along correct lines. A shoe which does these things should not be thought of as a corrective shoe but as a correct shoe.

A correct shoe for a growing child after walking begins should have the following construction (Figs. 48 and 49).

1. **Sole.** The sole should have a straight line on the medial aspect and a full, round toe to allow proper spread and freedom for the toes. It should be full across the ball as the child's foot is short and plump as compared with the adult foot and requires a greater proportionate width at this point. The sole should be firm enough to protect the foot but flexible in its forepart.

2. **Heel.** The heel seat and counter should be narrow so that it will grasp the os calcis and hold it firmly in posi-

tion. In sizes up to eight, the heel should be of the
wedge or spring type and from an eighth to three-sixteenths of an inch in height (Fig. 48C). In sizes over
eight, the heel should be the ordinary type and from
five-eighths to three-fourths of an inch in height (Fig.
49). The last over which the shoe is built, for reasons

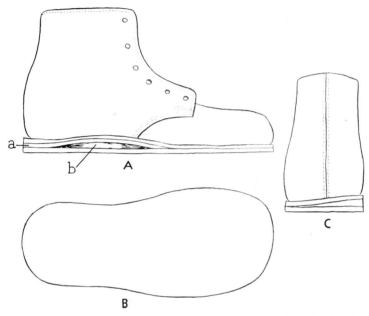

FIG. 48. The correct shoe for the growing child after walking begins. A, side
view showing the wedges of the sole which elevate the longitudinal arch; B, cut
of the sole gives ample toe room; C, rear view shows the tilting of the heel on the
medial side which overcomes pronation.

which will be discussed under the description of the
shank of the shoe, should be designed to allow the heel
to be one-eighth of an inch higher on the inner side
than on the outer side.

3. **Shank.** The shank of the shoe should not be broader
than the width of the foot. To provide adequate support
for the developing arch, the shank should be molded to
form a definite arch in the shoe. The highest point or
apex of this arch should not be under the scaphoid bone

but should be placed farther back under the anterior half of the os calcis so that this bone may be adequately supported on its medial side, and any tendency for the foot to roll inward and downward or pronate, prevented. If the last over which the shoe is made is designed so that the heel on the inner side is one-eighth inch higher than on the outer side, a much more effective molding of the

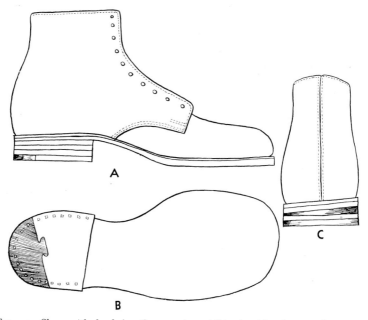

Fig. 49. Shoe with heel for the growing child. A, side view to show cut of upper and elevation of shank under the longitudinal arch; B, cut of sole gives ample toe room and slight extension of heel on the inner side gives support to the shank; C, rear view shows the tilt of the heel on the inner side which aids in overcoming pronation.

shank to form an arch is secured. In addition, sagging of the shank under the stress of use will be largely prevented. The shank of the shoe should be rigid. Rigidity in the shank is secured in the spring or wedge heel shoe by running two wedges of unequal length forward on the inner side of the sole (Fig. 48). The long wedge (a) elevates the medial side of the foot and tends to overcome pronation. The short wedge (b) molds the shank to form an arch. In the heeled shoe, rigidity is secured by incorporating in the leather shank a molded metal shank which runs from the middle of the heel seat to the ball of the shoe.

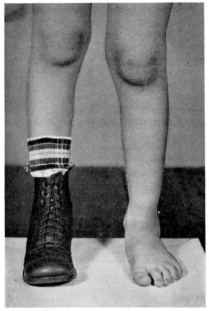

FIG. 50. A mild degree of pronation is shown in the unclothed foot; the amount of correction which can be obtained with a properly designed shoe is shown in the clothed foot. The correction of knock knee secured by balancing the foot is also shown.

4. **Upper.** In the small sizes, the upper should be of the high type reaching above the ankle and of blucher design. In the larger sizes, the oxford pattern of the upper will give ample support, but it should lace snugly over the instep and grasp it firmly.

A shoe with this construction fulfills the requirements necessary in a correct shoe and may be worn with advantage on a normal foot as well as on one showing postural faults (Fig. 50).

Rigid vs. Flexible Shank. As stated, there are many pediatricians and orthopedic surgeons who believe that a flexible-shank shoe should be worn by the growing child and that a rigid shank is to be avoided on the theory that the flexible shank permits freer movement, and hence, more normal development. With the claims made that the flexible type of shoe is superior because it allows greater freedom of movement in the toes and foot and so favors better muscle control of the growing foot, the authors cannot concur. Our observations and the observations of others have convinced us that in the growing foot, it is more important to maintain it in a balanced position on the leg than to build up muscle control. A flexible shoe will not hold the foot in a position of correct balance nearly as satisfactorily as will a shoe with a rigid shank, for, lacking rigidity, it adapts itself readily to the position the foot tends to assume instead of guiding it into the desired position of balance. The important part played by the muscles in maintaining foot balance is not disputed and should not be minimized; the effectiveness of muscle action, however, is very definitely dependent upon the integrity of the structural framework of the foot. Muscles alone cannot indefinitely hold an unbalanced foot in a position of balance any more than other muscles of the body can sustain indefinitely a constant contraction. It seems evident then that a balanced position of the foot must be established before effective muscle control can be built up. Moreover, we must not lose sight of the fact that today children carry out most of their activities on concrete sidewalks, brick playgrounds, and hardwood floors, and that under such conditions, the foot needs the definite protection which can be given only by a firm sole. It is, then, because experience has shown that a shoe with a rigid shank gives better protection for the growing foot and is more effective in holding the foot in a position of balance under conditions as they are today that it must be considered a better type of shoe both for the normal and for the abnormal foot of childhood than that which carries a flexible shank. Whether a rigid-shank shoe or one with a flexible shank is worn, it is imperative that the selection be made by a pediatrician or orthopedic surgeon, and not left to the discretion of a shoe salesman.

SUMMARY

The most important element in the care of the growing foot of childhood is that it be maintained in a position of balance. If structural strength is to be acquired, the foot must be allowed to grow and develop under conditions which insure an even distribution of weight stresses over the entire foot; unequal distribution of weight throws an increased burden on bones, ligaments, and muscles, and leads to disturbance in both structural and postural stability. Experience gained from years of observation indicates that in the growing child a correctly balanced shoe is the most reliable method of insuring that the foot will be maintained in balance and that exercises, while helpful, play a decidedly secondary role. The evidence, so far as the authors can determine, seems to favor the rigid type of shoe as best meeting the requirements of the child today.

7

FOOT IMBALANCE IN CHILDHOOD

In the preceding chapter the foot of childhood was discussed from the point of view of normal development. Not all growing feet, however, progress along correct lines of development. Many, for various reasons, are prevented from responding to the molding forces which should gradually shape them into efficiently working units or are subjected to distorting influences which tend to mold them into incorrect and weak forms, incapable of functioning properly and unable to meet the demands made upon them by growth and increasing activity. Broadly speaking, if, for any cause, a child's foot continues in its early position of pronation, normal development of its arches is made difficult or is prevented, and a weak or unbalanced foot results. The reasons for this seem quite clear when we realize that inrolling of the foot, or pronation, brings the thrust of the superimposed weight almost entirely on the medial side of the foot; this results in an improper concentration of weight stresses on the structures forming the longitudinal arch (bones and ligaments) and places undue strain upon the supporting and stabilizing muscles. When this unbalanced position of pronation persists in a growing foot beyond the time it should normally disappear, the foot is loosely termed a "flatfoot." That such pronated, unbalanced, or flat feet in children are not uncommon is recognized today by many pediatricians and by most orthopedic surgeons. Furthermore, it is an established fact that such foot imbalance is detrimental to the growing child, not only because of the foot strain and foot and leg tire which result, but also because it unquestionably influences unfavorably the attitude or posture of the entire body. Moreover, incorrect developmental tendencies in the growing foot have a strong proclivity to persist into adolescent and adult life with far-reaching effects upon the physical well being and efficiency of the individual. On these grounds, the importance of a study of the causes of imbalance in the growing foot of childhood and an understanding of the means of eliminating these causes at a time when the foot is most responsive to corrective measures, cannot be overestimated.

PREVALENCE

Reliable statistics on the prevalence of foot imbalance in children are not obtainable as hospital and private records rarely contain such information, at least not in usable form. In the authors' experience, in a fairly active hospital service and private practice, the incidence, in children, of foot imbalance sufficiently severe to produce symptoms has been relatively high. In a Boston hospital, it was stated some years ago that 44 per cent of the children seen in the outpatient department had some form of foot trouble. In an examination of 100 British school boys, it was revealed that 68 had deformities such as knock knee, bow leg, and flatfoot. In 1915, 25 per cent of all the children seen in the Orthopedic Outpatient Department of the Hospital of the University of Pennsylvania, had some form of postural defect; most of these cases had foot imbalance. No recent figures are available, but from those quoted, it is evident that in the past, foot defects in childhood were not uncommon, and it is certain that their prevalence has not decreased.

TYPES OF IMBALANCE

In the foot of a child, but one form of imbalance is common, and that is faulty lateral balance. Except in congenital club foot, infantile paralysis and spastic paralysis, the fault in lateral balance takes the form of pronation, or downward and inward rolling of the foot. In club foot, the fault in lateral balance is inversion of the foot or varus; in infantile paralysis or spastic paralysis, we may have either inrolling or outrolling, depending upon the muscle groups involved. We are concerned here only with faulty lateral balance of the postural variety; a discussion of foot imbalance due to infantile paralysis, spastic paralysis, and club foot does not fall within the scope of this book.

ETIOLOGY

Faulty lateral balance implies disturbance in both structural stability and postural stability. Any condition which interferes with the structural strength of the foot (arrangement of the bones and ligaments) or with the proper balancing of the leg on the foot (muscle control) becomes an etiologic factor in producing foot imbalance in childhood. Among the most common conditions responsible for foot imbalance in children are:

1. Muscle weakness.
2. Incorrect weight-bearing thrust on the foot owing to bow leg, knock knee, and tibial torsion.
3. Short heel cord.
4. Congenital defects, including a short first metatarsal bone, metatarsus varus primus, hypermobile first metatarsal segment, and accessory scaphoid.

Muscle Weakness

Weakness of the foot and leg muscles may be actual or relative; that is, there may be a true weakness or paralysis of the muscles which renders them incapable of performing their work properly; or the muscles may be normal in strength and power but, because of excess body weight, insufficient for the demands placed upon them. True muscle weakness may be the result of a condition of general asthenia, calcium and phosphorus deficiency (rickets), endocrine imbalance (usually thyroid or pituitary insufficiency), or infantile paralysis. Relative muscle weakness is, of course, as stated, due to excessive weight.

Muscle weakness from whatever cause becomes a factor in the production of foot imbalance when it results in the loss of lateral balance of the foot at the subastragalar joint, for it is through this joint that the balance of the foot in relation to the leg is maintained. Loss of control of this joint must result in faulty foot attitude and an unbalanced foot. If due to weakness of the pronators, the foot rolls outward at the subastragalar joint, the major part of the superimposed weight will fall on the lateral side of the foot (adduction). If due to weakness of the supinators, the foot rolls inward, the weight will fall on the medial side of the foot (pronation). In either circumstance, the foot is out of balance and unstable because of faulty muscle control. In the vast majority of cases, the foot assumes the position of pronation. This statement does not hold good in infantile paralysis, loss of muscle power due to nerve injury, or spastic paralysis, since in these conditions, the position the foot assumes will depend upon the muscle groups involved.

KNOCK KNEE AND BOW LEG

The body weight is distributed to the foot through the legs, the line of transmitted weight following the central axis of the tibia.

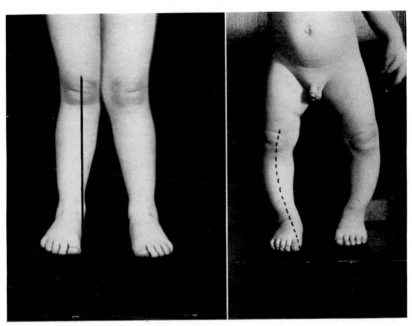

FIG. 51. Knock knee and bow leg. Note the line of weight concentration falls to the medial side of the foot.

The axis of the tibia is so nearly a straight line that a perpendicular dropped through the center of the patella will normally fall between the first and second metatarsal bones. In knock knee and bow leg, the axis of the tibia is not a straight line; in knock knee it angulates outward; in bow leg it curves outward and then inward. In both knock knee and bow leg, because the axis of the tibia deviates from an approximately straight line, the weight thrust on the foot is not transmitted directly downward but at an angle, and a perpendicular dropped through the center of the patella will fall toward the medial side of the foot through the first metatarsal or medial to it. The result of such shifting inward of the center of transmitted weight is to bring about an excessive concentration of the weight stresses on the inner side of the foot,

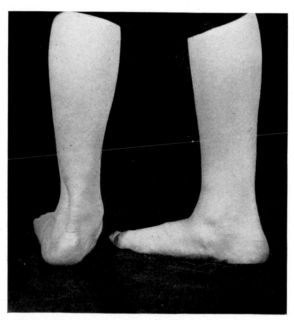

Fig. 52. Short heel tendon causing a downward and inward rolling of the foot at the subastragalar joint—pronation. The tendency of the short heel tendon to roll the os calcis inward is shown in the posterior view.

which rolls inward and downward or pronates with the usual sequelae that follow such an unbalanced position of the foot (Fig. 51). Torsion of the tibia to such an extent that the foot is everted or rotated outward around the central axis of the tibia produces the same faulty statics in the leg and foot as does knock knee or bow leg.

Short Heel Cord

A short heel cord affects the balance of the foot in two ways: First, shortness of the tendo achillis, since it lessens the arc of dorsal flexion, prevents acute flexion of the ankle so necessary to walking. As a result, when a step is taken, the forward progress of the leg can be continued only by a downward and inward rolling of the foot at the subastragalar joint; this exerts a depressing force upon the longitudinal arch. Second, shortness of the tendo achillis tends to roll the os calcis inward and tilt the subastragalar joint downward and inward (Fig. 52). This tilting in turn allows downward and inward rolling of the foot at the subastragalar joint, or pronation, and interferes with the development of the longitudinal arch of the foot.

Congenital Abnormalities of the Foot Bones

Shortness of Metatarsal I. The most common abnormality which occurs in the bones of the foot, as pointed out by Morton,

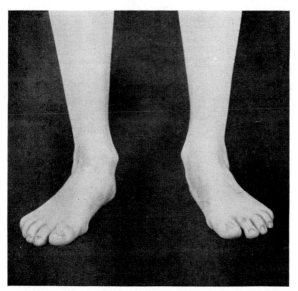

Fig. 53. Faulty foot balance, the result of a short metatarsal I and looseness of the first metatarsal segment. Fig. 53A, on page 86, x-ray of same foot.

is shortness of metatarsal I (Fig. 53). In the growing foot, its shortness brings about a definite disturbance in foot balance, which may have a profound influence on the development of the foot. Our observations have led us to conclude that if the first metatarsal is lacking in length, a definite amount of inrolling or pronation of the foot must take place in order that its head may come in contact with the weight-bearing surface, so that the position of pronation is habitually assumed (Fig. 53). In addition, since the head of the first metatarsal bone forms the anterior pier of the internal longitudinal arch, shortness of the first metatarsal lessens the stability of this important anterior buttress of the arch.

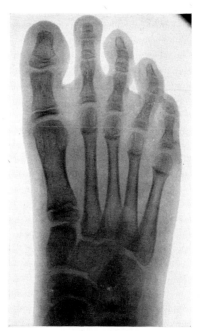

FIG. 53A. X-ray of foot shown in Fig. 53.

Hypermobility of the First Metatarsal Segment. Owing to laxness of the plantar ligaments of the first metatarsal segment (metatarsal I and medial cuneiform bones, Morton) there may be increased dorsal mobility of the first metatarsal bone. Its head thereby becomes less effective as a weight-bearing point because its lack of rigidity and stability permits inrolling or pronation. In other words, such hypermobility of the first metatarsal bones decreases the stability of the anterior pier of the inner longitudinal arch and allows pronation. If we have such hypermobility of the first metatarsal segment associated with a short first metatarsal bone, its effect is intensified (Fig. 53A).

Metatarsus Varus Primus. Metatarsus varus primus is an evolutionary deformity of the foot due to persistence of the prehuman position of the first metatarsal bone. The first metatarsal diverges from the second metatarsal and there is a wide separation of these

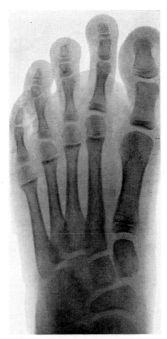

FIG. 54. Dorsiplantar x-ray of a child's foot showing metatarsus varus primus and hypermobility of the first metatarsal segment.

two bones which normally lie almost parallel. Metatarsus varus primus in our experience is usually associated with looseness of the first metatarsal segment, and there is consequently a definite hypermobility of the first metatarsal bone as well as a wide separation between it and the second metatarsal. The wide separation between metatarsals I and II and the greater mobility of the first metatarsal bone greatly diminishes the stability of the foot by lessening the stability of the anterior pier of the inner longitudinal arch. With impaired stability of the inner longitudinal arch, inrolling or pronation takes place (Fig. 54).

Accessory Scaphoid. Another fairly common bony abnormality which tends to cause an unbalanced position of the foot is

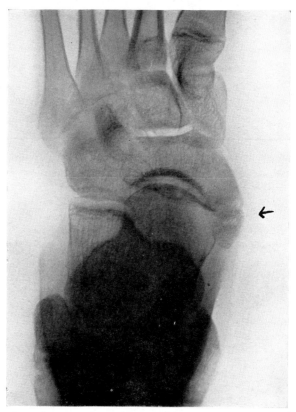

FIG. 55. Dorsiplantar x-ray of foot showing prehallux or accessory scaphoid.

prehallux or accessory scaphoid. An accessory scaphoid is a supernumerary bone, attached to or fused with the medial border of the scaphoid, which occasionally appears in the human foot (Kidner). When an accessory scaphoid is present, the tendon of the tibialis posticus, on its way to its final insertion in the internal cuneiform and metatarsals, is attached to the accessory bone instead of to the under surface of the scaphoid tubercle (Keith).

With this relationship, the tibialis posticus is forced to pull back-ward and inward at an angle and becomes a pronator instead of a supinator of the foot. Thus its lifting effect upon the longitudinal arch is reduced. It has also been noted that the prominence of the accessory scaphoid at times impinges on the internal malleolus and leads to discomfort to avoid which the foot is brought into a position of pronation (Fig. 55).

PATHOLOGY

As the result of improperly distributed weight stresses or be-cause of defective foot architecture, depression of the longitudinal arch and faulty alignment of the tarsal bones occurs in the un-balanced foot of childhood. Associated with such faulty alignment of the bones is stretching and relaxation of the supporting liga-ments. The essential pathology is then a loss of the compact arrangement of the tarsal bones so essential to satisfactory func-tioning of the foot as a support for the body and as a propulsive lever in locomotion.

SYMPTOMS

Subjective. The subjective symptoms of foot imbalance in the growing child are few. Indeed, there may be no subjective symp-toms complained of which point directly toward the foot. Usu-ally the child is brought for examination because the mother has noticed that it has an awkward gait or "toes in" or "toes out," rather than because of any complaint of discomfort on the child's part. The most consistent complaints are that the child tires un-duly, is disinclined to do much walking, and that the legs pain at night—sometimes erroneously spoken of as "growing pains." "Growing pains" as such do not exist, and leg pains in a child are the expression of muscle strain and tire—the result of incor-rect statics in the legs and feet.

Objective. The examination of the feet for objective evidence of foot imbalance should be conducted with the child both stand-ing and sitting in order that a complete evaluation of the condi-tions present may be made.

The standing examination should be made with the child

stripped, at least from the waist down, and placed on an elevated platform facing the examiner with the feet pointed forward parallel to each other, and about three inches apart. Inrolling or pronation, absence of the normal longitudinal arch, and prominence of the scaphoid bone indicate faulty foot balance (Fig. 56).

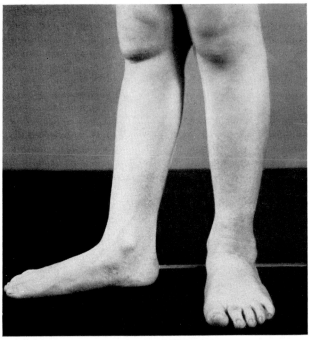

Fig. 56. Faulty foot balance in the child; showing pronation, depressed longitudinal arch and prominence of the scaphoid.

The child should then be turned with his back to the examiner and, if pronation is present, prominence of the internal malleolus and an inward tilting of the heel will be evident. If the heel cord is short or tight, the tendo achillis will be displaced to the lateral side of the ankle (Fig. 52).

The alignment of the foot and leg should be checked. In children, muscle weakness, knock knee, bow leg, and torsion of the tibia are the most common causes of malalignment of the foot on the leg. When deformity of the leg bones is present, it is worth while recording the amount of distortion for reference later in checking the improvement. The amount of knock knee present can be estimated fairly accurately by measuring the distance between the internal malleoli with the child standing and the knees in contact; the amount of bow leg by measuring the distance between the medial condyles of the femora, the crests of the tibia, and the internal malleoli, with the child standing and the medial sides of the feet in contact. Torsion of the tibia can be estimated by placing the legs side by side with the patella pointing forward and noting the amount of outward or inward rotation of the foot with reference to a plane passing through the middle of the patella.

With the child in a sitting position, a very careful examination of the entire foot should be made for the purpose of determining the condition of the ligaments, muscles, bones, and circulation. This inspection should include a determination of the tone of the ligaments (whether they are of normal tone or relaxed), the presence of weakness or paralysis of muscle groups, or interference with muscle balance, and whether any abnormality of the foot bones is present. The heel cord should always be tested for shortness. If the tendo achillis is short, it will be difficult to dorso-flex the foot to an acute angle or even to a right angle with the knee extended and the foot moderately adducted.

After examination of the child in standing and sitting position, the gait should be observed. The usual tendency of the pronated foot in walking is to "toe out," the foot being held in an everted or abducted position. Intoeing, however, is not infrequent; this position of the foot is probably a compensatory measure adopted unconsciously. Intoeing should be looked upon as an encouraging sign and a definite effort on the part of the child to overcome the unbalanced position of the foot.

X-RAY

As a rule, the x-ray gives little information about the foot of a child, but if any abnormality of the foot bones is present or suspected, an x-ray should always be made. The plate should be taken in the dorsiplantar plane in weight-bearing and with the feet parallel.

If there is any marked degree of pronation, it is advisable to make a pedograph for record (Fig. 57).

DIAGNOSIS

The diagnosis of imbalance in the foot of a child is based to some extent on the subjective symptoms indicating foot strain but mainly from the objective findings obtained by a careful foot examination. The outstanding objective findings may be listed as

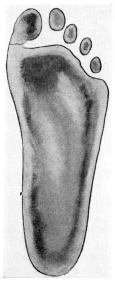

FIG. 57. Pedograph of a child's foot with pes planus.

pronation, lack of normal longitudinal arch, short heel cord, leg deformities, and congenital abnormalities of the foot bones. The x-ray is particularly helpful in determining the presence of abnormalities of the foot bones and should be made use of more freely than it has been in the past.

TREATMENT

The underlying pathology of foot imbalance in childhood is: (1) Locally, a disturbance of structural (bones and ligaments) and postural (muscle) stability in the foot; and (2) generally, any constitutional condition which tends through its effect upon the ligaments, bones, and muscles to cause weakness in these structures. Since causes may be both local and general, treatment must be planned along both local and general lines.

LOCAL TREATMENT

The objective aimed at by local treatment is to convert an unbalanced foot into a balanced one and maintain it in its balanced position.

PRONATION

Since pronation is the primary fault in the unbalanced foot of childhood, overcoming pronation is the first step in treatment. In mild cases, correction of pronation is accomplished by clothing the foot in a properly designed shoe of the type already discussed (page 73, "Foot of Childhood"). If, however, the shoe does not entirely correct pronation, the foot may be rolled outward and the longitudinal arch elevated by placing in the shoe an inlay or support. The most efficient support in the authors' experience is an oval-shaped inlay made of hard piano felt, one-fourth of an inch in thickness on its inner side and skived or beveled to the front, back, and outer edges as shown in Fig. 58. The support should be so placed in the shoe that the highest point on the inner side will lie well back under the sustentaculum tali of the os calcis and not forward under the scaphoid bone. In this position the support exerts an upward thrust against the sustentaculum tali and prevents inrolling of the os calcis and depression of the subastragalar joint and effectively corrects pronation. If, after the addition of such a support, pronation still persists, the heel of the shoe should be elevated or wedged one-eighth to three-sixteenths of an inch on the inner side (Fig. 59). Wedging the heel in this manner will tilt the shoe outward and elevate the medial side of the foot sufficiently, as a rule, completely to overcome pronation unless it is extreme or the individual is excessively heavy. Occasionally, it may be necessary to elevate the inner margin of the sole of the shoe as well as the heel. This, however, is seldom required and is, as a rule, undesirable since, when the entire inner

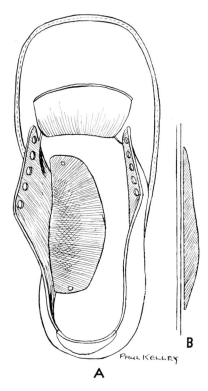

Fig. 58. The placement of an oval support in a child's shoe to overcome pronation. B, side view of support to show contour.

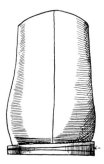

Fig. 59. Rear view of a child's shoe showing the heel wedged on the inner side to overcome pronation.

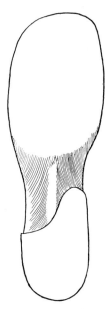

FIG. 60. Thomas or extension heel gives added support to the shank of the shoe.

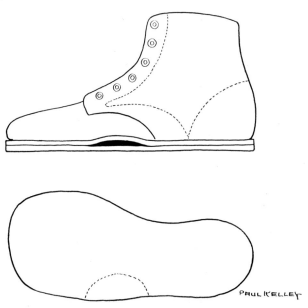

FIG. 61. Position of metatarsal wedge on the outer side of the sole.

side of the shoe is elevated, the foot tends to slide over to the outer side of the shoe and away from the support instead of rolling outward, and the effectiveness of the support is lessened. In very heavy children, who have reached the age at which a heeled shoe is worn, it may be necessary to use an extension or a Thomas heel to prevent the shank of the shoe giving way under the burden of excessive weight and allowing the foot to roll inward (Fig. 60). It is usually advisable, if the inner side of the heel has been elevated, to wedge the outer side of the sole one-eighth of an inch at a point opposite the head of the fifth metatarsal (metatarsal wedge) (Fig. 61). This prevents the forepart of the foot from sliding outward in the shoe and enhances the effectiveness of the support under the longitudinal arch.

SHORT METATARSAL I, HYPERMOBILE FIRST METATARSAL SEGMENT, METATARSUS VARUS PRIMUS

If a short metatarsal I, hypermobile first metatarsal segment, or metatarsus varus primus is present, a platform approximately three-sixteenths of an inch thick should be placed under the head of the first metatarsal bone as suggested by Morton (Fig. 62). This platform may be made of hard felt or sponge rubber. Such a platform acts by establishing proper contact between the head of metatarsal I and the supporting surface, a contact which is impossible with a short first metatarsal or an excessively movable one, such as we have with a hypermobile first metatarsal segment or metatarsus varus primus. By establishing a proper contact between the head of metatarsal I and the supporting surface, the anterior pillar of the inner longitudinal arch is stabilized and pronation is minimized. Also, it seems reasonable to expect that if a short metatarsal I is compelled to do its proper share of weight-bearing by the use of a platform it may, in the growing foot, respond to the stimulation of use by increasing in length and in time become normal, and that a hypermobile first metatarsal segment in time may become more stable. If this result can be accomplished, a most important step toward the prevention of permanent foot imbalance will have been taken.

ACCESSORY SCAPHOID

An accessory scaphoid, if pronounced enough to be a definite factor in foot imbalance, should be removed and the tendon of the tibialis posticus muscle be given a new attachment (page 134).

KNOCK KNEE, BOW LEG, TIBIAL TORSION

Correction of knock knee and bow leg and tibial torsion is necessary if pronation is to be overcome. Such distortion of the

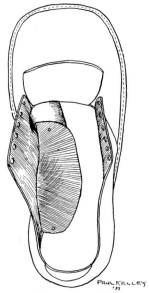

FIG. 62. Placement of metatarsal platform with oval inlay.

leg bones results in a concentration of weight stresses on the inner side of the foot and favors inrolling or pronation. Further-more, pronation of the foot tends to increase the deformity al-ready present or prevent its correction and a vicious circle is established. The principles governing the correction of bow leg and knock knee are identical. The problem to be dealt with is one of a faulty line of transmitted weight, which tends to become more exaggerated under the stress of weight-bearing. We know that bones adapt themselves in form, structure, and alignment to meet the demands which stresses make upon them. If, then, we desire to change the form and alignment of deformed leg bones, such as are found in bow leg, knock knee, and tibial torsion, we must alter the lines of stress in such a way as to influence them to grow away from deformity and toward the normal. Any device which will roll the foot outward and elevate its inner margin will alter the direction of the line of weight-bearing, lessen the deforming stresses upon the leg bones, and tend to influence their

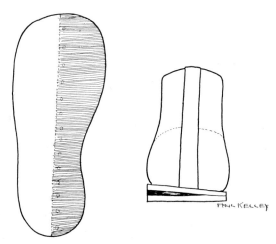

FIG. 63. The sole and rear view of a child's shoe showing the position of the wedge on the inner side of the heel and sole used in the correction of bow leg and knock knee.

growth toward a straight line from knee to ankle. Outward rolling of the foot in both bow leg and knock knee is brought about by placing a wedge one-eighth to three-sixteenths of an inch thick on the inner side of both the heel and sole of the shoe in addition to the felt support under the longitudinal arch (Fig. 63). In bow leg, balancing the shoe in this manner apparently increases the deformity, yet it actually corrects it. We are aware that many physicians and even some orthopedic surgeons raise the outer side of the shoe in treating bow leg. Such a procedure is wrong and serves only to accentuate inward rolling of the foot, thus depressing the already low longitudinal arch, augmenting deforming stresses and favoring increasing deformity. When balancing a shoe to correct bow leg, it is usually advisable to place a metatarsal wedge in the outer side of the sole of the shoe opposite the head of the fifth metatarsal bone (Fig. 61). Such a metatarsal wedge prevents outward sliding of the foot in the shoe and prevents outward torsion of the forepart of the foot on the posterior part of the foot; torsion strain between movable posterior and fixed posterior parts of the foot is a definite feature of pronation owing to bow leg because of the manner in which the weight stresses are transmitted to the foot.

SHORT HEEL TENDON

Shortness of the heel tendon provides a very definite obstacle to overcoming pronation. A child's foot should flex dorsally and inward to at least 80 degrees. If it can be flexed dorsally and inward only 90 degrees or more, the heel tendon is short, and it must be stretched or lengthened if pronation is to be corrected. Such stretching or lengthening may be accomplished in one of two ways:

1. The child may be put on heel-stretching exercises.
2. The heel tendons may be stretched and the foot placed in a plaster cast.

The logical line of procedure is first to attempt to stretch the short heel cord by exercises. The purpose of the exercises should be explained to the mother to obtain intelligent co-operation, and both parent and child should be carefully instructed in the exercises prescribed. Exercises useful in elongating a contracted heel cord will be found in the chapter on "Exercises."

If, after a reasonable trial of exercise treatment, the heel tendon fails to respond, manual stretching of the short heel cord followed by the application of a plaster cast should be carried out.

Manual Stretching of a Short Heel Cord. Anesthesia should not be used. The child is placed on a table in the recumbent position and the knees flexed to about a right angle. The foot is then grasped well back toward the heel and brought forcibly into dorsal flexion and adduction. This manipulation is repeated until the foot can be dorsiflexed to 90 degrees or better in the adduction position. A cast is then applied from below the knee to the ends of the toes with the foot in as much dorsal flexion and adduction as possible; the cast is bi-valved (Fig. 64). At the end of a week

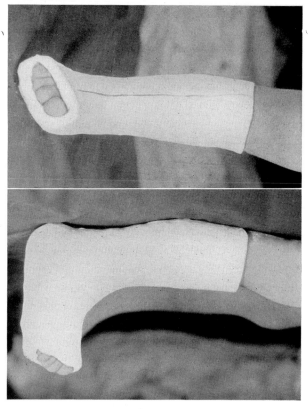

FIG. 64. Heel tendon stretched and held in the corrected position by a plaster cast. Side view is shown at the top, the toe view below.

or ten days, the cast is removed, the stretching repeated, and a cast applied which is allowed to remain on the foot another week or ten days. After the second cast is removed, the foot will, as a rule, dorsally flex in adduction to 80 degrees. Heel-stretching exercises should be carried out daily for several months. It is best not to attempt to secure too much correction of the foot by the first manipulation, as discomfort and unnecessary suffering may be caused. This is avoided by dividing the stretching into two stages. Manipulation with anesthesia frequently leads to overdoing the stretching, and discomfort and even actual suffering result; it is for this reason that stretching is more satisfactory without an anesthetic.

EXERCISES

Exercises are of unquestionable value in the treatment of functional foot disorders. In young children, unfortunately, it is quite difficult to have exercises properly and systematically carried out, and in the very young the main reliance must be placed in the proper balancing of the foot. With older children, exercises should be used to develop both the intrinsic muscles of the foot and the muscles of the leg in order that they may function at maximum efficiency in supporting the arches and maintaining the best balance of the foot on the leg. A description of the exercises used will be found in the chapter on "Exercises."

CONSTITUTIONAL TREATMENT

Overweight, disturbance of the endocrine glands, and calcium and phosphorus deficiency are the most common general conditions which play a part in the production of foot imbalance in children. Overweight in childhood is a distinct factor in the causation of an unbalanced foot in that it throws an excessive burden upon the immature foot and makes difficult its development along normal lines. Disturbance of the endocrine glands acts in two ways: First, by producing overweight; and, second, apparently by influencing in ways not yet understood the development of the osseous system; certainly, in some cases, endocrine imbalance seems to be responsible for the development of such deformities as bow leg, knock knee, and tibial torsion. Our clinical experience, at least, has been that in a definite percentage of cases leg deformities have been found associated with stigmata of endocrine imbalance. Calcium and phosphorus deficiency are unquestionably the underlying cause in most cases of knock knee and bow leg, and so such deficiency must be considered a very definite contributing factor in the production of foot imbalance.

Simple overweight should respond to careful dietary measures, but co-operation of both the patient and the parents is necessary for success. In all obese children, careful search should be made for the symptoms of endocrine imbalance, which may be hypothyroidism or hypopituitarism or both. In properly selected cases, the use of fairly large doses of thyroid or the hypodermic administration of pituitary extract, anterior or posterior lobe, or a combination of these, will often result in astonishing improvement, not only in the physical condition but also in the mental make-up and the response of the child. Thyroid and pituitary therapy, however, must be used under strict supervision and with due regard to the indications for its use based on a careful study of the child.

Calcium and phosphorus deficiency manifest themselves in muscular weakness and bone deformity (knock knee, bow leg, and tibial torsion). When calcium and phosphorus deficiency is present, purposeful measures should be taken to increase the fixed calcium and phosphorus. Cod-liver oil and sunlight or, failing this, the ultraviolet ray are still our main reliance for increasing the utilization of calcium. In our clinical experience, cod-liver oil has been more effective than the irradiated sterols, and we advise its use in tablespoonful doses three times a day after meals. Recent laboratory investigation seems to support the clinical evidence as to the greater efficiency of cod-liver oil. Natural sunlight is preferable to artificial rays, but if the latter are used, the best wave lengths are about 300 millimicra.

SUMMARY

Foot imbalance in childhood is comparatively common. Correction of faulty foot balance in childhood is important because of the unnecessary strain and consequent tiring which result and because of the unfavorable effect which it has upon general posture. Correction in childhood of faults in foot balance is also important because it can be accomplished more easily at this time than in later life as the foot is in a more plastic state and its structure is more readily altered (Fig. 65). It should be recognized that failure to correct faulty foot balance in childhood may later

lead to much unnecessary discomfort and disability, for such faults
tend to persist into adolescent and adult life and cause functional

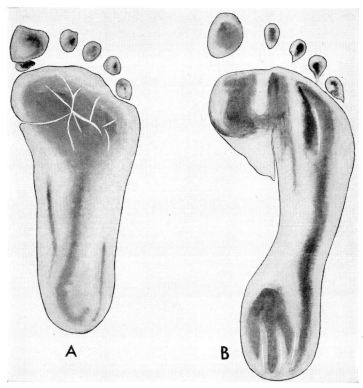

FIG. 65. Pedographs of a child's foot. A, before treatment showing marked pes
planus or flatfoot; B, same foot after three years of treatment (shoes, supports and
exercises).

foot disorders which give rise to discomfort and suffering and
even serious incapacity.

8

FOOT IMBALANCE IN ADOLESCENCE

The preceding chapter dealt with foot imbalance in the growing child, a period which may be considered to extend from the time the child begins to walk until the age of eight or ten years has been reached. From this time up to the age of eighteen years is the adolescent period. The adolescent period is a very important one in foot development as the bones, muscles, and ligaments have become fully matured, and the foot is beginning to "set," as it were, in its permanent form. If, in the growing foot of childhood, all deforming factors have been eliminated, the individual should arrive at the adolescent period with a balanced foot, which, while it may not be perfect, should be satisfactory from the point of view of function. If, however, because of neglect or ignorance, or in spite of earnest attempts to overcome foot faults, the individual enters the adolescent period with an unbalanced foot, the situation may be described as serious without being guilty of overstatement. The seriousness of the situation lies first in the fact that correction of faulty foot attitude by conservative measures is far more difficult in the more mature foot of adolescence than it is in the developing foot; and, second, unless faults are corrected, they will be carried on into adult life and may seriously handicap the physical efficiency of the individual. Stated in another way, after the adolescent period has been reached, the foot begins rapidly to lose its plastic character and responds less readily to forces which in the more malleable stage of its development may be used effectively to correct faulty architecture and mold the foot into a more efficiently functioning organ; but it still provides more satisfactory material for plastic alteration than does the even more rigid foot of the adult. Viewed in this way, it should be evident that this important period in the development of the foot demands thoughtful attention, and its discussion is perhaps the most important material to be presented. Dismissing the problem of foot imbalance in the adolescent as of no moment is assuming a serious responsibility, as it so often results in a lost opportunity really to correct faulty foot attitude and may condemn the individual to a future of discomfort and limitation of physical activity. The views here presented are based upon years of experience and continuous observation; and, while possibly

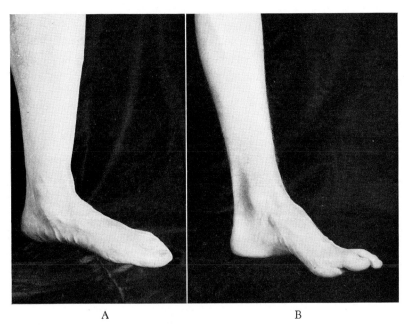

A   B

Fig. 66. Foot imbalance in adolescence. A, pes planus or flatfoot; B, pes cavus or high-arched foot.

they may be at variance with those held by others with equally wide or greater opportunities for observation, they represent the authors' conclusions and state their position.

TYPES OF FOOT IMBALANCE

Whereas in the foot of the growing child we are concerned only with faulty lateral balance, that is, pronation and depression of the longitudinal arch, in the more developed adolescent foot, we find in addition to faulty lateral balance, faults of anterior-posterior balance. Faults in anterior-posterior balance involve the anterior or metatarsal arch and are usually, in the adolescent foot, the result of an abnormally high not a low longitudinal arch. We have, then, in the adolescent foot two basic types of foot imbalance:

1. A low-arched foot, pes planus or flatfoot (Fig. 66A).
2. A high-arched, adducted foot with contracted plantar fascia and prominent ball, or pes cavus (Fig. 66B).

There is, as well, an almost infinite variety of combinations of these two basic types. It seems wise, however, in the interest of clarity, to discuss only these two types.

Adolescent Flatfoot
(Pes Planus)

ETIOLOGY

All that has been said under etiology in discussing pes planus or flatfoot in the growing foot of childhood holds good for the adolescent foot. The same causative factors which bring about inrolling or pronation of the foot and depression of the longitudinal arch in childhood are responsible for pes planus in the period of adolescence. They are:

1. Muscle weakness.
2. Incorrect weight-bearing thrust on the foot owing to knock knee, bow leg, and tibial torsion (Fig. 67).
3. Short heel cord.
4. Congenital or developmental defects involving the bones of the foot (short first metatarsal, hypermobile first metatarsal segment, metatarsus varus primus, and accessory scaphoid) (Figs. 68-69).

The way in which these conditions cause pronation of the foot and depression of the longitudinal arch has already been discussed in detail in the chapters on "Primary Causes of Foot Imbalance" and "Foot Imbalance in Childhood." It should suffice here to mention only in a general way the manner in which each becomes a factor in the production of functional foot disorders in the adolescent.

Muscle weakness or loss of muscle balance between the pronator and supinator groups results in the loss of lateral balance of the foot at the subastragalar joint with pronation or supination of the foot—usually the former. Incorrect weight-bearing thrust owing to knock knee, bow leg, or tibial torsion brings about an excessive concentration of weight stresses on the inner side of

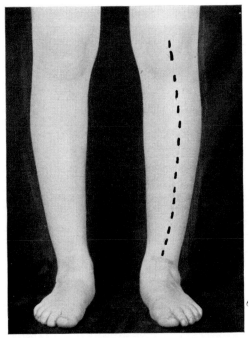

FIG. 67. Pronation of the feet in adolescence owing to tibial torsion and bowing

the foot and causes downward and inward rolling of the foot or pronation. A short heel cord necessitates a downward and inward rolling of the foot at the subastragalar joint in walking, and tends to tilt the os calcis inward; the effect of this malalignment of the astragalus and the os calcis is to cause pronation or depression of the longitudinal arch. A short first metatarsal bone, relaxation of the first metatarsal segment, and metatarsus varus primus lessen the stability of the anterior pier of the inner longitudinal arch, allowing foot to pronate and longitudinal arch to descend.

PATHOLOGY

The pathology present is a malalignment of the tarsal bones and ligamentous relaxation; this results in the loss of the normal,

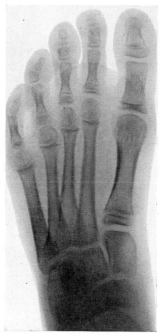

Fig. 68. Dorsiplantar x-ray of foot showing short metatarsal I and hypermobile first metatarsal segment.

compact arrangement of the bones composing the foot arches. With a short first metatarsal bone, hypermobile first metatarsal segment, and metatarsus varus primus, there is concentration of weight stresses on the second metatarsal bone, which enlarges. Evidence of such hypertrophy of the second metatarsal, in response to the increased burden thrown upon it, begins to appear in the adolescent foot (Fig. 70).

SYMPTOMS

Subjective. The symptoms complained of are those which result from ligamentous strain and muscle tire. The most common subjective symptoms are tiring and pain in the feet. Tiring is usually complained of in the longitudinal arch, on the inner side of the foot; pain is most commonly localized in the region of the scaphoid bone owing to irritation of the subastragalar joint. With

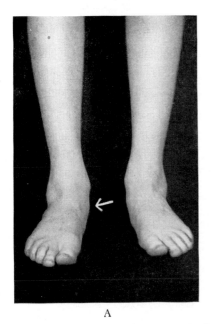

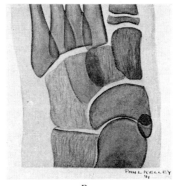

A   B

Fig. 69. Prehallux or accessory scaphoid. A, patient showing marked pronation and prominence of the scaphoid bones; B, dorsiplantar x-ray showing accessory scaphoid.

a short first metatarsal bone, pain is sometimes complained of on the plantar surface at the base of the second metatarsal bone because of irritation of the joint between it and the middle cuneiform bone (Fig. 71). In addition to the symptoms in the foot itself, there is often leg ache owing to tiring of the leg muscles through their effort to overcome the postural instability present. General tiring or exhaustion after what should be a normal amount of activity and disinclination to activity are often complained of. Such a series of complaints should always suggest inspection of the foot for objective evidence of foot imbalance.

Objective. The routine of a complete foot examination has been given in Chapter 5, and the details need not be repeated here. For general inspection of the foot, the child should be

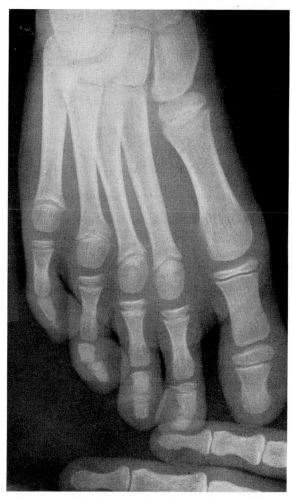

Fig. 70. Dorsiplantar x-ray of adolescent foot showing short metatarsal I and hyper-trophy of metatarsal II and mild degree of metatarsus varus primus.

stripped, at least up to the waist, and placed on an elevated plat-form, standing facing the examiner and with the feet parallel and about three inches apart. In this position, any malalignment of the legs, such as bow leg, knock knee, and tibial torsion will at once be evident. Pronation or inward and downward rolling of the foot, absence of the normal longitudinal arch, and prominence of the scaphoid bone indicate a flatfoot (Fig. 72). The child should then stand with his back toward the examiner with

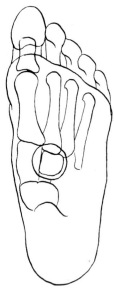

Fig. 71. Drawing of sole of foot; circle indicates localization of pain in foot imbalance.

the feet in the same position. Prominence of the internal malleolus and inward tilting of the heel, if present, will confirm the diagnosis of flatfoot. Displacement of the heel cord toward the lateral side of the ankle suggests a short heel cord (Fig. 73).

One should examine for shortness of the heel cord. The presence of a short heel cord is determined by dorsally flexing and adducting the foot with the knee extended. If the foot does not dorsally flex to at least 85 degrees, the heel cord is short.

Definite shortness of the great toe implies a short metatarsal I. Wide separation of the first and second toes with hypermobility of the first metatarsal segment indicates that metatarsus varus primus is present. Undue prominence of the scaphoid suggests the possibility of an accessory scaphoid.

The presence of callosities and corns is a definite indication that the weight-bearing is faulty and that imbalance is present.

X-Ray Evidence. While the x-ray perhaps affords little information in the average unbalanced adolescent foot, when pos-

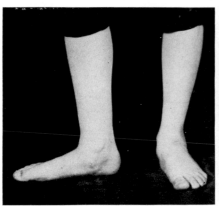 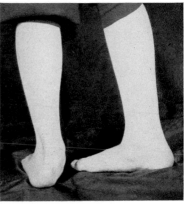

Fig. 72   Fig. 73

Fig. 72. Pes planus in adolescence. Note pronation, depression of longitudinal arch, and prominence of the scaphoid bone.

Fig. 73. Pes planus in adolescence (rear view). Note pronation, prominence of the internal malleolus, and lateral displacement of the heel cord.

sible, a skiagram should be made; an x-ray of the foot should be insisted upon if a short first metatarsal, metatarsus varus primus, or accessory scaphoid is suspected. Increase in the size of the second metatarsal bone makes its appearance during the adolescent period and can be seen in an x-ray film (Fig. 70). Overdevelopment of the second metatarsal bone is an evidence of increased concentration of weight upon the head of this bone and that the first metatarsal bone is not performing its share of the work either because it is short or hypermobile. Metatarsus varus primus is present when there is medial divergence of the first metatarsal bone, a wide interspace between the first and second metatarsals, and a tendency on the part of the great toe to divert laterally and assume a hallux valgus position. Hypermobility of the first metatarsal segment is indicated by an increased degree of separation between the medial and middle cuneiform bones (Fig. 74). Plates should be taken in the dorsiplantar position in weight-bearing.

The evidence upon which a diagnosis of flatfoot or pes planus in the adolescent is made is essentially the same as that for flatfoot in the growing child. The only difference between the un-

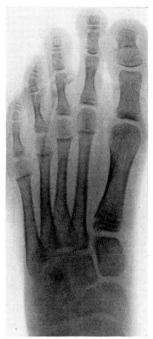

Fig. 74. Dorsiplantar x-ray of an adolescent foot showing separation between the medial and middle cuneiform and hypermobility of the first metatarsal segment.

DIAGNOSIS

balanced foot of childhood and that of adolescence is that in the latter the subjective symptoms become more important and the objective findings more pronounced. The unbalanced adolescent foot usually shows more evidences of faulty balance in the form of corns and callosities, particularly over the head of the second metatarsal bone and over the tuberosity of the fifth metatarsal bone. X-ray studies are more important than in the growing foot, as the effect of abnormal weight distribution on the bones of the foot first becomes evident in the adolescent period.

TREATMENT

The decision as to what form of treatment should be carried out in the management of adolescent foot imbalance is often an important one, since the result of treatment may have a far-reaching influence upon the future welfare of the individual. The primary purpose of treatment in the adolescent period should be correction of faults in balance, not merely securing symptomatic relief. Correction of faulty foot attitude should insure the individual going into and probably through adult life with satisfactorily functioning feet. Failure to correct faulty foot balance makes highly probable a future of foot discomfort, limitation of physical activity, and continuous wearing of arch supports of one kind or another. The treatment of the unbalanced foot of adolescence should, then, be undertaken from a different point of view than that held toward the developing foot of childhood already discussed. In childhood, only conservative methods of treatment, designed to guide the growing foot along correct lines of development, are indicated; in the adolescent foot, which has to a large extent lost its plastic qualities, less is to be expected from conservative treatment and operative measures may be necessary to overcome postural faults which have become so set as to be resistant to conservative methods of correction. In the adolescent, then, the treatment of foot imbalance may follow two lines: conservative and operative.

Conservative Treatment. Unquestionably, conservative measures should be our main reliance in the treatment of adolescent foot disorders, and such conservative measures should be persisted in until it is evident that satisfactory results cannot be obtained by their use. The period of time during which conservative measures are justified depends upon the behavior of the foot under treatment and the extent to which the causative factors respond. Conservative treatment may properly extend over a period of years or may be terminated after a much shorter period of trial if no real improvement is shown. Certainly there can be no justification for continuing routinely to balance shoes and prescribe arch supports for an adolescent flatfoot which has evident structural faults and which does not show any indication of improvement under treatment. Such methods merely carry the individual on into adult life unimproved, and the future holds nothing for him but a continuation of the same form of treatment. For example, it is proper treatment in an adolescent pes planus due to a short heel cord to prescribe correct shoes and adequate supports and to employ exercises to stretch the heel tendon. It is not proper treatment to persist in such measures if the short heel tendon is not lengthened and the foot imbalance is not corrected by such conservative measures. Stretching the heel cord by manipulation or lengthening of the heel cord by operation under such circumstances is not only indicated but imperative if the foot faults are to be overcome and a real cure consequently obtained.

Conservative measures have as their objectives the following: (1) Correction of inrolling or pronation and descent of the arches of the foot; (2) stimulation of growth in a short first metatarsal bone, if this is possible, and overcoming relaxation in a hypermobile first metatarsal segment, if this can be accomplished, by bringing the foot into proper position of balance; (3) correction of such structural faults in the leg as short heel cord, knock knee, bow leg, and tibial torsion.

Pronation and descent of the longitudinal and transverse arches is best overcome by the use of a correct shoe, properly balanced to meet the conditions present, and supplying an adequate support for the arch.

SHOES. The best shoe for the adolescent foot is one which will give efficient support and yet does not depart so far from the lines of style that the shoe will be objectionable. The average girl in the adolescent period is becoming style conscious, and if a shoe with extreme lines is forced upon her an attitude of antagonism toward the treatment will be aroused, co-operation will be lacking, and there will be, in all probability, little benefit derived from treatment. The ideal shoe or oxford for the adolescent is one built on a straight last with a moderately round toe; such a shoe will afford ample room for free action of the toes and yet will have enough style in the fore-shoe to be attractive (Fig. 75). The upper should be of a blucher or bal type and should lace snugly over the instep. The shank should be moderately broad, that is, as broad as the waist of the foot, and should, to provide firmness, be reinforced by a steel shank, extending from

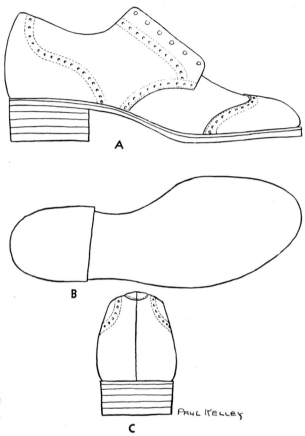

FIG. 75. Growing girl's oxford. A, side view to show cut of upper; B, view of sole which gives ample toe room. Heel is extended slightly on the inner side to give added support to the shank. C, rear view of heel.

the heel to the ball of the foot. The heel seat and counter should fit snugly around the heel to hold the foot in correct position. The height of the heel in the growing girl's shoe should be twelve-eighths or one and one-half inches high until the size of two or three is required, when the adult heel of twelve-eighths or fourteen-eighths inch is correct. The height of the heel in the boy's shoe will vary from five-eighths to an inch. A shoe of this type provides a satisfactory foot covering for the normal foot and serves as an excellent foundation for such additions as may be necessary to bring about balance in an unbalanced foot.

SUPPORTS. Arch supports are designed to elevate both the longitudinal and metatarsal arches to approximately their proper position. Arch supports are of two types: (1) rigid supports, made of metal, celluloid, or composition; (2) nonrigid supports, made of leather, hard felt, or sponge rubber. Of the rigid type of support, the Whitman foot plate, made of metal fashioned over a cast of the foot, is best. A description of the Whitman foot plate will be found on page 164. Whatever the advantage of a metal support in treating pes planus in the adult, it is not, in the authors' opinion, suitable for treatment of the adolescent foot; nonrigid supports are, as a rule, to be preferred, for they are more comfortable, less traumatizing, and just as effective.

AUTHORS' NONRIGID SUPPORT.—The authors' nonrigid supports are described in detail in the chapter on "Foot Imbalance in the Adult." Here the molding and application of these supports will be discussed in a rather general way to avoid unnecessary repetition.

The support is made of sponge rubber of fairly firm consistency. It has been found most satisfactory to have the support manufactured in the rough by rubber manufacturing companies, for they can be furnished in bulk at a very low cost. The support has two parts: a longitudinal section for the longitudinal arch, and an anterior section for the metatarsal arch (Fig. 76). The longitudinal section is approximately one-fourth inch thick on the inner side at its high point and tapers to a feather edge on the outer side and posteriorly. Anteriorly, it is somewhat bevelled and gradually merges into the anterior section to support the metatarsal arch. The anterior section of the support is rounded into shape to conform approximately to the line of the heads of the metatarsal bones; the height at its anterior margin is about three-sixteenths of an inch (Fig. 76C). Such a roughly molded support can be readily shaped to the proper height for both the longitudinal and metatarsal arches by using a sharp knife, or better, by grinding on a rough emery wheel. The support should extend from just posterior to the head of the second metatarsal bone to well back under the heel. The high point of the longitudinal section of the support should lie under the anterior one-third of the os calcis, i.e., under the sustentaculum tali, not

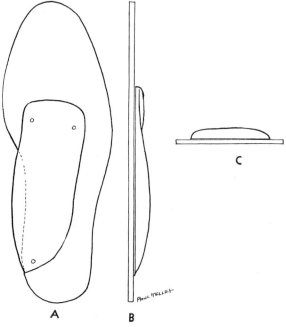

Fig. 76. Support used in the treatment of pes cavus. A, position of support on insole; B, side view of support showing contour; C, anterior view of support.

forward under the scaphoid bone. When the high point of the support lies under the sustentaculum tali, it exerts a thrust against this bony projection which rotates the os calcis outward; this counteracts the tendency of the subastragalar joint to roll downward and inward and brings the foot bones into their proper relationship with each other. If the high point of the longitudinal support is placed under the scaphoid bone, it elevates the arch by a direct upward thrust against the superimposed weight and does not utilize the mechanics of the arch itself to bring about correction of faulty foot attitude; in other words, it attempts to jack the foot up by main force. The anterior section of the support is made whatever height may seem necessary to give adequate support to the metatarsal arch.

When the support has been fitted and fashioned to the desired form, it is placed in the shoe and firmly fastened. The exact

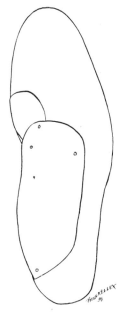

FIG. 77. The position of the first metatarsal platform as used in combination with the longitudinal arch support.

position of the support is determined by measuring the distance from the head of metatarsal II to the back of the heel with a caliper. This caliper distance is used to locate the inlay by placing one point of the caliper flush with the counter of the heel, when the other caliper point will indicate the head of metatarsal II and, therefore, the position of the anterior end of the support. In fastening the support into the shoe, it is best to use two or three shoe tacks. Large headed carpet tacks should not be used. After being placed in position, the support should be covered with thin leather or leather substitute, both of which can be obtained from any shoe supply house at small cost.

A short metatarsal I should be elevated by a platform or support placed under the head of the first metatarsal bone in addition to the support for the longitudinal arch. The platform may be made of sponge rubber or felt; it should be three-sixteenths of an inch high and fixed firmly to the insole of the shoe in the proper position under the head of the first metatarsal bone (Fig. 77). Metatarsus varus primus and hypermobile first metatarsal segment require the same type of balancing by support and plat-

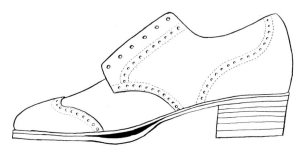

Fig. 78. Position of metatarsal wedge on the outer side of the sole.

form. The details of the construction and placing of a platform will be found on page 175.

Frequently, alterations in the heel and sole of the shoe are necessary correctly to align a foot which is out of balance. Wedging the inner side of the heel one-eighth to three-sixteenths of an inch is often necessary to overcome pronation which is not corrected by the shoe and an inside support. It is generally advisable to place a wedge one-eighth inch in thickness and approximately one and one-half inches long in the sole of the shoe opposite the head of the fifth metatarsal bone to prevent the foot sliding outward in the shoe and to align the bones of the fore-part of the foot with the posterior part (Fig. 78). If weight is excessive, an extended or Thomas heel adds greatly to the supporting qualities of the shank of the shoe and aids in preventing pronation (Fig. 79).

A short heel tendon may be stretched by the intensive use of heel stretching exercises, or it may be stretched manually and the foot and leg placed in a plaster cast. If, in the adolescent, these conservative measures fail to relax the heel tendon and careful observation indicates that the short heel cord is a definite obstacle to overcoming pronation, the heel tendon should be lengthened by operation. Heel stretching exercises are discussed in the chapter on "Exercises." Manual stretching of a short heel cord is described in the chapter on "Foot Imbalance in Childhood."

Knock knee, bow leg, and tibial torsion should be corrected by conservative measures if possible. Correction of knock knee, bow leg, and tibial torsion is favored, during the period of growth,

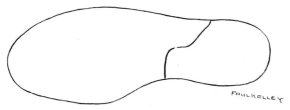

FIG. 79. Thomas or extension heel gives additional support to the shank.

by altering the weight-bearing stresses on the leg bones so that as they grow they will tend to change their direction from an angular or rotated plane between the knee and the ankle to an approximately straight line between these two points. This alteration in weight stresses is brought about in both knock knee and bow leg by placing a wedge on the inner side of the shoe, both heel and sole, one-eighth to three-sixteenths of an inch high and a support inside the shoe to roll the foot outward exactly as is done in the foot of the growing child. Tilting the foot outward shifts the line of transmitted weight away from the medial toward the lateral side of the foot and brings a corrective stress on the deformed leg bones. If knock knee, bow leg, and tibial torsion persist, notwithstanding long continued conservative treatment, and if the distortion of the leg bones is sufficient to nullify efforts to overcome the unbalanced position of the foot, correction of the deformity by operation is indicated. Operative correction of knock knee, bow leg, and tibial torsion should not be advised, however, until conservative measures have been thoroughly tried out and unless there can be no question but that the deformity is the cause of failure to get results. In our experience, it is seldom necessary to resort to operative correction of knock knee, bow leg, and tibial torsion in the adolescent.

Operative Treatment. By far the majority of functional foot disorders in the adolescent period should be treated conservatively; there are, however, certain adolescent feet which are so defective because of fundamental faults in architecture or mechanics that correction by conservative measures is impossible. An unbalanced foot of the latter type presents a very definite problem, for, unless the faulty foot attitude is corrected before adult age is reached, the individual can only look forward to a continuation of discomfort, interference with normal activity, and a lifetime of treatment in the effort to secure foot comfort. Faults in foot balance which do not respond to well-planned conservative treatment can often be improved by surgery, and a few operations, designed to correct faulty architecture or faulty mechanics, have been accepted by orthopedic surgeons. Faced with the failure of conservative measures to bring about real correction in a symptom-producing foot, the patient should be given an opportunity to enjoy the benefits to be derived from a soundly planned and properly performed operation. The operative treatment of foot imbalance, however, requires experience and judgment and should be attempted only by those with a wide experience in foot mechanics and thoroughly familiar with the technic of the procedure to be carried out. The results of operations on the feet, at least those of a stabilizing type, are permanent and final. Great harm may follow failure to bring the foot into proper alignment at the time of operation, so that the outcome is a disaster to be regretted for all time.

Operative procedures useful in overcoming faulty foot attitudes which are responsible for functional foot disorders are of three types: (1) Those which are carried out for the purpose of lengthening or relaxing contracted structures which prevent the foot from assuming a position of balance; (2) those designed to reinforce the ligaments important in maintaining the integrity of the

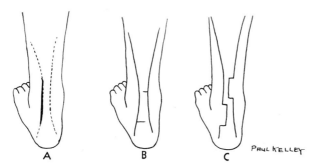

FIG. 80. Technic of lengthening heel tendon. A, line of incision; B, position of transverse incisions in tendon; C, the lengthened heel tendon.

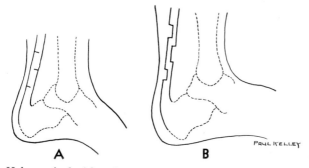

FIG. 81. Hoke method of lengthening heel tendon. A, position of transverse incisions in the heel tendon; B, heel tendon lengthened.

arch; and (3) arthrodesing operations on the foot joints for the purpose of correcting architectural faults in the foot which cannot be corrected by ordinary conservative measures or less drastic forms of operation. Lengthening of a short heel cord and lengthening of a contracted plantar fascia are examples of the first type; an operation described by Charles S. Young, which utilizes the anterior tibial tendon to reinforce the first medial tarsometatarsal ligament and the plantar navicular-cuneiform ligament, is an example of the second type; the Hoke and Miller flatfoot operations are examples of the third type.

OPERATIVE LENGTHENING OF A SHORT HEEL CORD. This operation is indicated when, notwithstanding a conscientious trial of exercise and manual stretching, the heel cord remains contracted or shortened sufficiently to be a definite factor in causing pronation or inrolling of the foot with depression of the longitudinal arch.

The technic of the operation is briefly as follows. The heel cord is exposed by a longitudinal incision approximately three inches long placed one-half inch lateral to the tendo achillis (Fig. 80A). The skin is dissected back and the entire width of the tendon is exposed. A longitudinal split is then made in the tendon sheath which is reflected, exposing the tendon itself. Increased length of the tendon may be secured by incising of the tendon at different levels and strongly dorsiflexing the foot, when the tendon will elongate the desired length by the two sections gliding past each other.

Incisions made in the tendon to permit this gliding may be placed in various ways. A simple method is one in which an incision carried two-thirds of the distance across the tendon is made near the insertion of the tendon into the os calcis, and a second incision made on the opposite side of the tendon about three inches proximal to the first, also carried two-thirds of the distance across the tendon (Fig. 80B-C).

Hoke has described a method in which three incisions are used: two transverse incisions on the superior surface of the tendon about three inches apart, and a single transverse incision on the inferior surface about midway between these two incisions, or slightly toward the distal cut (Fig. 81). The tendon sheath is not opened in the Hoke procedure; the incisions pass through the tendon sheath and into the tendon. The foot is now strongly dorsiflexed and the tendon lengthened longitudinally to the desired length.

There are other types of incisions which may be used, but these two methods are satisfactory and simple; the authors prefer the Hoke method. In closing the incision, the tendon sheath should be carefully approximated with a fine catgut suture if it has been opened. The skin may be closed in whatever manner the operator prefers.

After the incision is closed, a cast extending from the ends of the toes to the tibial tubercle is applied with the foot in the desired amount of dorsiflexion. The cast is worn for two to three weeks, after which time walking may be resumed gradually. In lengthening the heel tendon, care should be taken to avoid too much relaxation or mild calcaneus will develop and walking be interfered with. This operation may be performed at any time after the age of six or eight years.

THE YOUNG OPERATION FOR THE TREATMENT OF PES PLANUS. Charles S. Young has described an operation for the correction of pes planus. He states that this operation is applicable to cases of pes planus in which the deformity is not rigid and in which there are no arthritic changes in the intertarsal joints.

TECHNIC. A lengthening of the tendo calcaneus is performed as a preliminary procedure so that the anterior end of the calcaneus can be elevated when the arch is raised. The tendon should be divided by a long oblique incision and lengthened so that dorsiflexion of the ankle is limited only by the posterior ligament of the ankle joint. In the operation on the foot itself, a slightly curved incision with convexity upward is made on its medial aspect from the shaft of the first metatarsal bone to the inferior extremity of the medial malleolus. The incision should pass superior to the medial aspect of the navicular bone. After reflecting the skin and superficial fascia, the larger branches of the medial

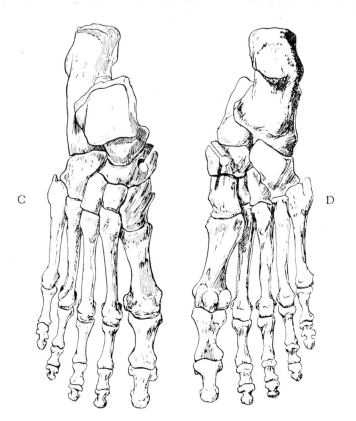

C   D

FIG. 81, C and D. Operative treatment of pes planus. (Charles S. Young, M.D.) C, Skeleton of the right foot from the superior aspect, showing position of drill hole and slot in the navicular bone. D, Plantar view illustrating drill hole and slot from this aspect. Attention is called to the shaded area which indicates the groove on the inferior surfaces of the navicular and first cuneiform bones.

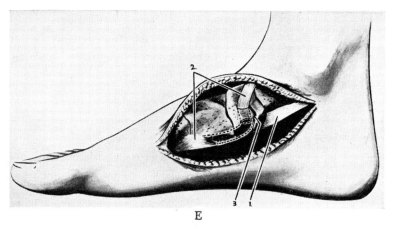

E

FIG. 81E. Operative treatment of pes planus. (Charles S. Young, M.D.) The tendon of the tibialis anterior muscle is looped through a drill hole in the navicular bone. (1) Tendon of tibialis posterior. (2) Tendon of tibialis anterior. (3) Slot from drill hole to posterior part of medial aspect of navicular bone.

tarsal artery in the region of the superior aspect of the navicular bone should be exposed under the deep fascia and ligated. The tendon of the tibialis posterior muscle is temporarily separated with a periosteal elevator from its attachment to the inferior surface of the navicular tuberosity. The medial one-half of the inferior surfaces of the navicular and first cuneiform bones are exposed. A drill hole 6 mm. or 7 mm. in diameter is made vertically through the navicular bone, lateral to the tuberosity from the superior to the inferior surface. The superior opening of the drill hole is made oval in shape with a gouge. A slot 2 mm. wide is made with a gigli saw and very thin chisel from the drill hole to the posterior part of the medial surface of the navicular tuberosity (Fig. 81C, D). A small gouge is used to make a groove on the inferior surfaces of the first cuneiform and the navicular bones from the insertion of the tibialis anterior muscle to the drill hole at its inferior end. The sheath of the tibialis anterior tendon is exposed and incised in its distal 6 or 8 cm. After freeing the tendon down to its insertion, it is pulled posterior with a button hook and thrust through the slot in the navicular bone to a position in the drill hole, and in the groove on the inferior surfaces of the navicular and first cuneiform bones (Fig. 81E). Two pronged instruments in the shape of the letter U on the end of a rod are useful to force the tendon through the slot. The small chips of bone taken from the slot are replaced. No retentive sutures are necessary, because the tendon is firmly fixed in its new position. The tendon of the tibialis posterior is replaced as near as possible to its original position.

Following the operation, the extremity is immobilized with a plaster cast from the toes to the upper part of the thigh. The ankle is fixed in its limit of dorsiflexion and the knee in twenty degrees of flexion. The sutures are removed through a window in the cast two weeks postoperative. The cast is removed seven or eight weeks after the operation to allow firm healing of the tendo calcaneus. Obviously, the operation on the foot itself would require immobilization only a short time after the incision has healed. When walking is started, the lateral side of the heel of the shoe should be lowered one-eighth to one-fourth of an inch, to prevent eversion strain, for six months or longer in some cases. Resistive exercises should be given daily in this interval to develop the tibialis anterior and tibialis posterior muscles.

COMMENT. This operation raises the arch of the foot by adding the power of the tibialis anterior muscle to that of the tibialis posterior near the point of primary insertion of the latter on the navicular bone. The tension on the tendon of the tibialis anterior from the position of its insertion, to the inferior opening of the drill hole in the navicular bone, makes it act as a ligament in that part of its changed course. It reinforces the first medial tarsometatarsal ligament and the plantar navicular cuneiform ligament and in that way helps to prevent depression of the arch and abduction of the forefoot. The physiologic effect of the operation is so to balance the muscle power of the foot that the weight of the body is sustained by the bones of the arch without strain on the ligaments and muscles. Postural tonus of the muscles is all that is required to maintain this balance.

This operation should not be applied until after the age of ten years, because prior to that age ossification has not progressed sufficiently in the tarsal navicular bone. If performed before the navicular bone is largely ossified, it is necessary to use a mattress suture of heavy chromic catgut to bind the two surfaces of the slot in the bone together.

The authors have used this procedure a number of times, and have found it satisfactory in correcting persistent pronation without excessive depression of the arch. It has not proved so satisfactory where marked depression of the arch was present with a well-established pes planus.

STABILIZING OPERATIONS FOR THE CORRECTION OF PES PLANUS. A variety of arthrodesing operations have been suggested to overcome pes planus and do away with the necessity of wearing supports. Such arthrodesing operations find their greatest field of usefulness in the adolescent and young adult. They should be used with caution in those over thirty. So far as the adolescent foot is concerned, a stabilizing operation is indicated when the foot is

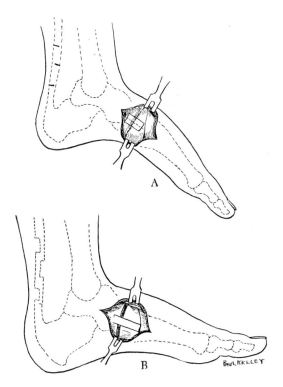

FIG. 82. Hoke flatfoot operation. A, the transverse incisions in the heel tendon for lengthening; exposure of the scaphoid-cuneiform joint; outline for the rectangular section of bone cut from the scaphoid and internal cuneiform. B, the position of the bones, the graft, and the lengthened heel tendon when the operation is finished.

extremely flat and relaxed and shows no indication of improvement with conscientiously carried out conservative treatment. Stabilizing operations should not be performed before the age of twelve or fourteen years of age. Two stabilizing operations are commonly used and are of proved worth; these are the Hoke and the Miller operations for the correction of pes planus.

HOKE FLATFOOT OPERATION. The first step in the operation is lengthening the contracted heel cord; this may be done by any one of the accepted methods. Thereafter, in the operation the assistant holds the foot in equinus by grasping the ball of the foot and forcibly pressing the foot into a cavus position. A linear incision is then made over the medial aspect of the scaphoid-cuneiform joint. The incision is carried down to the bone and periosteal flaps are dissected back, exposing the scaphoid-cuneiform joint. With a thin osteotome, cutting deeply, the cartilage surfaces of the contiguous parts of the scaphoid, internal and middle cuneiform bones are removed. A rectangular section of bone one-half inch deep is cut from the scaphoid and internal cuneiform bones (Fig. 82A). The pieces are taken out and cut into bits. A bone graft the size of the rectangle is taken from the tibia and driven into the rectangular receptacle (Fig. 82B); the bits of bone are packed into the deep and superficial spaces not filled by the graft. The periosteal flaps are closed over the graft. The incision is closed by layers and thin dressings are applied. The foot is held in an equinus cavus position and a plaster splint is molded on the foot. The splint is molded well under the scaphoid-cuneiform joint and, just before it hardens, the posterior end of the heel is twisted inward. After the splint has hardened, the edges of the plaster shoe are turned up and padding inserted underneath them. The foot is then dorsiflexed so that it makes a 90-degree angle with the leg. The plaster shoe prevents any change in the bony relationship in this angle. The cast is completed to the midthigh.

Two weeks after the operation, the cast, dressings, and skin sutures are removed. The foot bones are maintained in their position and a cast is applied from the toes to the tibial tubercle. At the end of six weeks, the cast is removed and the foot is fitted in a properly designed shoe with a rigid shank. It is advisable to carry some support under the elevated arch for some months following operation.

THE MILLER FLATFOOT OPERATION. A linear incision is made along the medial side of the tarsus from a point over the neck of the astragalus forward over the bodies of the scaphoid and internal cuneiform bone and ending at the base of the first metatarsal bone.

The subcutaneous fascia is dissected up and the insertion of the anterior and posterior tibial tendons identified. With a thin osteotome, a flap including the insertion of the calcaneoscaphoid ligament and the posterior tibial tendon is lifted up with a thin slab of bone from the sides of the scaphoid and internal cuneiform bones; this is held back with a retractor (Fig. 83A). This exposes the joints between the astragalus and scaphoid and the internal cuneiform and the base of the first metatarsal bones. The lesser articular ligaments are lifted upward and downward subperiosteally and preserved as well as possible to reapply over the area of fusion. The articular surfaces between the scaphoid and internal cuneiform and internal cuneiform and first metatarsal bone are resected with a thin osteotome (Fig. 83B). If the heel cord is short or contracted, it is lengthened at this stage.

The forefoot is now manipulated into adduction and the first metatarsal rotated into a corrected position. With the foot held in adduction the flap containing the calcaneoscaphoid ligament, the insertion of the posterior tibial tendon and the slab of bone are pulled forward under tension and transplanted as a graft to the body of the internal cuneiform bone and base of the first metatarsal (Fig. 83C). This whole mass passes forward beneath the anterior tibial tendon which is not disturbed at its insertion. The wound is closed in layers.

A plaster boot is applied with the foot in the corrected position. At the end of six to eight weeks, the cast is removed and the foot fitted in a supporting shoe. An inlay or support should be worn in the shoe for some months to preserve the corrected position while the fusion is consolidating.

Both of these operations have proved satisfactory in the hands

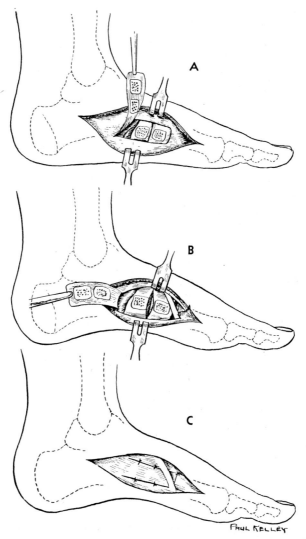

FIG. 83. Miller plastic flatfoot operation. A, showing fascia dissected up with slab of bone from side of scaphoid and internal cuneiform bones; B, the articular cartilage between scaphoid, internal cuneiform and base of first metatarsal bones has been excised (note the slab of bone lifted with periosteum from side of first metatarsal); C, showing the fascia sutured in place maintaining a normal arch line.

of experienced operators. In the opinion of the authors, the Hoke procedure, which is less extensive than that of Miller, gives excellent results in younger individuals and where the pes planus is not extreme. The Miller operation has been more effective in older individuals with marked pes planus.

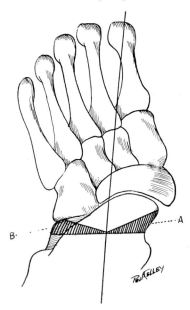

Fig. 83D. White's operation for congenital flatfoot. (A) Wedge removed from the astragalar neck to shorten the medial border of the foot. (B) Opened-up osteotomy in the os calcis into which the wedge of bone from the neck of the astragalus has been introduced to lengthen the lateral border of the foot. (Redrawn from *The Journal of Bone and Joint Surgery.*)

WHITE'S OPERATION FOR CONGENITAL FLATFOOT. J. Warren White describes an operation for the correction of congenital flatfoot too severe for conservative therapy. The pathology upon which the technic described is based is an elongation of the neck of the astragalus, resulting in elongation of the inner border of the foot and shortening of the outer border. The purpose accomplished by the operation is shortening of the inner border of the foot and lengthening of the outer border. This latter, White feels, is necessary for complete correction of the valgus deformity.

The operation is performed as follows: A two-inch longitudinal incision is made over the medial border of the foot, centered over the neck of the astragalus. The neck of the astragalus is exposed and cut completely across with an osteotome to a point where the body and neck join. A second cut is made with the osteotome, beginning three-eighths to one-half inch anterior to the first osteotomy, directed backward to contact the end of the first osteotomy about in the middle of the foot, a quarter to one-half inch lateral to the medial extremity of the first osteotomy. The result of this procedure is removal of a wedge-shaped portion of the neck of the astragalus (Fig. 83D). A third osteotomy is then made across the calcaneus; the line of this osteotomy is about one-quarter of an inch posterior to the calcaneocuboid joint and in a line with the astragalar osteotomy on the medial side of the foot. This osteotomy of the os calcis emerges on the medial side of the foot just anterior to the forward end of the sustentaculum tali. The fore part of the foot is now swung inward, closing the wedge in the astragalar neck and opening up a wedge on the lateral surface of the calcaneum. The wedge of bone removed from the astragalus is placed in the wedge-shaped opening in the calcaneum and trimmed flush with its surface. If more correction is desired, because of the inaccessibility of the astragalar neck, the overhanging navicular tuberosity may be chiseled off, and a wedge ranging up to twice the width at the base may be excised. Both wounds are closed in layers and a plaster-of-Paris cast applied from just below the knee to the ends of the toes with the fore foot in as much varus as can be easily obtained and in slight equinus.

If the heel cord is short, it should be lengthened as a preliminary step. White has found this necessary in about one-half the cases.

The cast is worn for two months. After its removal, a shoe wedged one-eighth of an inch on the inner side of the heel is worn for six months. Exercises directed toward mobilizing the foot and strengthening the tibial group of muscles are started immediately after removal of the cast. White reports satisfactory results in seventeen out of eighteen cases.

KIDNER'S OPERATION FOR FLATFOOT DUE TO ACCESSORY SCAPH-OID. When depression of the longitudinal arch is due to faulty action of the posterior tibial tendon because of its insertion into an accessory scaphoid or prehallux instead of into the undersur face of the scaphoid bone, F. G. Kidner has suggested the follow ing operation.

The incision follows the course of the posterior tibial tendon with its center placed at the prominence of the prehallux. The tendon is freed upward for one and one-half inches. Below, it is freed for one-half inch by an artificial dissection of the fibers going to the cuboid and metatarsals. With an osteotome, a thin layer of bone is cut off the prehallux, thus freeing the tendon. Next, a piece of bone which includes the whole prehallux in cases where the bone is free or a corresponding amount of the scaphoid if it is fused, is removed. More bone is removed below than above. The tendon with its thin sliver of bone is then trans planted downward so that it is in contact with the freshly cut undersurface of the scaphoid. It is held in this position by two or three chromic sutures to the adjacent ligamentous tissues. This transplantation is carried out with the foot in almost full supination. The wound is then closed by layers and the foot is put up in a plaster cast in full supination with a moderate amount of cavus. Fixation is maintained for six weeks and then physio therapy is started with gradual return to weight-bearing in a supporting shoe with a slight wedge on the inner side of the heel. It is advisable to place a support inside the shoe to maintain the corrected position until the posterior tibial muscle is functioning satisfactorily.

HIGH-ARCHED FOOT
(PES CAVUS)

ETIOLOGY

An abnormally high arch in a foot is largely a congenital condition; at least, a tendency toward the development of a high-arched foot becomes evident quite early in life. Asso ciated with a high-arched foot in the adolescent are shortness of the heel cord, contraction and thickening of the plantar fascia, and a tendency to equinocavus deformity. In some cases, the faulty architecture of the foot seems to be responsible for the shortening of the heel cord and plantar fascia. In other cases, shortening must be looked upon as the cause of pes cavus, although the underlying condition which causes the shortening of these structures is not always clear. It is possible that the contracture of the heel cord and plantar fascia may be a throwback in development to the pronograde type of foot. In the

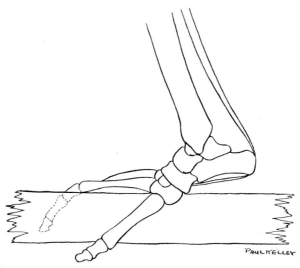

FIG. 84. Pronograde type of foot. Note the continuity of the plantaris and the plantar fascia. (After Keith.)

pronograde animal, the tendon of the plantaris muscle passes over the heel to combine with and help the plantar fascia; a persistence of part of this anatomic relationship may explain the occurrence of a pes cavus—in some cases at least (Fig. 84). Pes cavus also occurs as the result of muscle imbalance, due to infantile paralysis and spastic paralysis.

SYMPTOMS

Subjective. The high-arched foot is, as a rule, less likely to cause painful symptoms than a flatfoot. A pes cavus is not a weak foot but a rigid one, and while it lacks elasticity, it bears up under the stress and strain of use quite well, at least until fairly late in life. In the high-arched foot, the disturbance is mainly one of anterior-posterior balance and the major part of the burden of weight-bearing is borne by the anterior part of the foot, the metatarsal heads; consequently, the usual symptoms are pain and discomfort in the ball of the foot and callus formation over this region. At times there is pain in the longitudinal arch, especially after excessive use, and occasionally pain is complained of in the calf muscles due to tiring of these muscles from toe walking or strain on the short heel cord. Often, however, there are no subjective complaints, and advice is sought because it is difficult to get a shoe which fits satisfactorily.

Objective. For examination, the same position should be assumed as for any foot examination; that is, with the patient standing on an elevated platform with the feet parallel and about three inches apart.

With the patient facing the examiner, it will be seen that the longitudinal arch is not depressed but quite high. The forepart of the foot is usually adducted or "toes in," and the line of transmitted weight is shifted toward the lateral side of the foot (Fig. 85). In brief, the attitude of the foot is just the opposite of that which is characteristic of pes planus. Inrolling of the foot may be present, but such inrolling takes place at the joint between the tibia and the astragalus and is not a true pronation.

With the patient seated and with the foot relaxed, the ball of the foot is prominent, and there is often beginning callus formation over the heads of the metatarsal bones. In the more advanced cases, the toes are contracted into a hammertoe position, and corns over the phalangeal joints may be present. The plantar fascia is usually contracted—often so much so that it stretches across the arch of the foot very much like the string of a tight bow (Fig. 86). The heel cord is found to be actually shortened or is functionally short by reason of the dropping down of the forepart of the foot owing to the elevation of the longitudinal arch.

TREATMENT

While the necessity for treatment in the adolescent high-arched foot is perhaps not so urgent as is that of pes planus, still it is important. If the faulty attitude is not corrected, symptoms will appear later in life and interference with normal physical activity will eventually occur. The treatment of pes cavus in the adolescent, as in pes planus, should aim at correction of fundamental defects

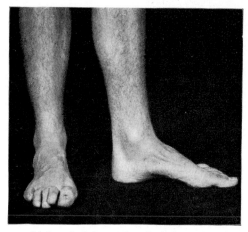

FIG. 85. Pes cavus or high-arched foot. Note high longitudinal arch and the tendency of the foot to roll to the lateral side.

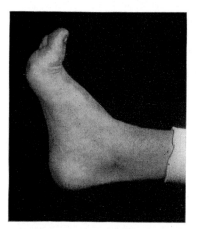

FIG. 86. High-arched foot with prominence of the ball and contracted plantar fascia.

present and not merely seek to relieve symptoms. Such correction may be secured by conservative measures, but occasionally operative interference is necessary.

Conservative Treatment. Conservative treatment should be planned: (1) to balance the foot so that the entire foot will function in weight-bearing and not merely the anterior part; (2) to overcome contraction of the plantar fascia, shortness of the heel cord, and contractures of the toes. The foot is balanced by using a correct shoe, and in addition supplying a support which will properly distribute the body weight over the entire foot. Contraction of the plantar fascia is often overcome by elevating the depressed forepart of the foot through proper balancing of the shoe. The short heel cord and contracture of the toes are best overcome by exercises.

SHOES. The type of shoe recommended for use in pes planus is also suitable for the high-arched foot. This is a shoe with straight lines on the inner side, a moderately rounded toe, a moderately wide shank reinforced with a steel arch, a well-fitting heel counter, and a heel fourteen-eighths inches to sixteen-eighths inches high for girls and five-eighths inches for boys. As a rule, the only shoe alteration required satisfactorily to balance a high-arched foot is a metatarsal wedge one-eighth of an inch thick and one and one-half inches in length placed in the outer side of the sole of the shoe opposite the head of the fifth metatarsal bone. A metatarsal wedge prevents the foot from sliding outward in the shoe, tends to overcome the adduction of the forepart of the foot and brings it into better alignment with the posterior part of the foot, and, finally, tends to shift the line of transmitted weight toward the medial side and away from the lateral side of the foot.

SUPPORTS. Supports useful in the correction of pes cavus may be of the rigid type (metal) or nonrigid type (felt, celluloid, or sponge rubber). It is the authors' opinion that in the adolescent foot the nonrigid type of support is best because it is less harsh to the foot and more resilient. The sponge-rubber support described on page 117 for use in adolescent flatfoot, may be used with some modifications for the treatment of pes cavus. Supports for a high-arched foot should be designed to bring about a proper

ratio of weight distribution over the entire foot. To do this, the
entire sole of the foot must be brought into contact with the
weight-bearing surface, not merely the anterior part. This is accomplished by placing under the longitudinal arch a support of
sufficient height to fill in the space between the shank of the shoe
and the elevated longitudinal arch which, as a rule, is so high that

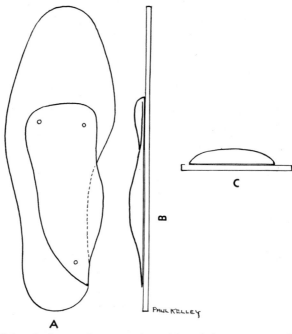

FIG. 87. High-arched type of support. A, position of the support on the insole; B,
side view showing contour of the support; C, anterior view of support.

it has no contact with the shank of the shoe. In modeling the
longitudinal section of the support for the high-arched foot, the
highest point of the support should lie under the scaphoid bone
and not under the sustentaculum tali, for this type of foot does
not require to be rolled outward as does the flatfoot (Fig. 87).
The longitudinal section of the support should be prolonged
forward under the metatarsal bones to elevate them and relieve
the metatarsal heads of the excessive burden thrown upon them.
As a rule the height of the anterior section of the support is

greater than that used in the treatment of pes planus in order that the metatarsal heads may be elevated sufficiently to avoid excessive pressure on them. Such a support with an elevation under both the metatarsal and longitudinal arches relaxes the plantar fascia, brings the entire sole of the foot in contact with the bearing surface, and so insures that the entire foot will take part in weight-bearing.

As the heel cord is nearly always short, actually or relatively, except in paralytic cases, heel-stretching exercises should be employed to overcome the shortening. Occasionally, stretching by manipulation and the application of a plaster cast may be advantageously used to bring about lengthening or stretching of a short heel cord which does not respond to exercises.

EXERCISES. Since the toes in most cavus feet are contracted into a more or less hammertoe position, marble or jack exercises may be used to advantage to elevate the ball of the foot and straighten out the contracted toes. These exercises as well as those used for stretching a contracted heel tendon, are discussed in the chapter on "Exercises."

Occasionally the combination of high-arched foot and inrolling of the ankle joint is encountered. Such a combination presents a difficult problem and one which can be met only by such balancing of the foot as will place it in the best weight-bearing attitude.

Conservative treatment thoroughly supervised and conscientiously carried out over as long a period of time as necessary will in the vast majority of cases bring about a satisfactory remodeling of the adolescent high-arched foot and will insure that, with reasonable care, discomfort and impairment of function in later life will be prevented.

Operative Treatment. Operative measures play a much less important role in the management of adolescent pes cavus than they do in pes planus and should be used with caution.

Elevation of the heel is nearly always present in pes cavus, but lengthening of the tendo achillis by operation is rarely if ever indicated. The reason for this lies in the fact that elevation of the heel is not in many cases a real elevation brought about by a contracted heel tendon, but is an apparent elevation due to the dropping downward of the forepart of the foot. This dropping down of the forepart of the foot is due to the abnormal elevation of the longitudinal arch which causes a malalignment of the foot bones and the assumption of an equinocavus position. Lengthening of the heel cord under such circumstances can only result in still further elevation of the longitudinal arch by allowing the os calcis to drop downward into a position of calcaneus with disastrous results. Lengthening of the heel tendon in the cavus foot, then, may be said to be indicated only when there is an actual shortening of the heel cord to an extent which is seriously interfering with the correction of the faulty balance present.

From time to time, an adolescent pes cavus is seen in which the contracture or thickening of the plantar fascia is so extreme that correction by conservative means is impossible (Fig. 86). If, after a reasonable trial of conservative measures, progress is unsatisfactory or no improvement is evident, lengthening of the plantar fascia by operation is indicated. A contracted plantar fascia should never be tenotomized as recurrence of the contracture is common; relaxation of plantar fascia should be secured by a stripping of the os calcis as described by Steindler.

STEINDLER'S OPERATION. A linear incision is made on the medial side of the heel extending from the inner tubercle of the os calcis forward for about two inches. Dissection is carried down between the layers of fat and the plantar surface of the plantar fascia, entirely exposing the plantar fascia from its insertion on the os calcis forward for two inches. The fascia is then incised crosswise close to the point where it blends into the lower surface of the os calcis. The muscles covered by the plantar fascia are medially to laterally, the abductor of the great toe, the short flexors of the great toe, and the abductor of the fifth toe. The muscles are now stripped off the periosteum of the os calcis with a blunt instrument, extending the stripping forward to the calcaneal-cuboid junction in order to reach and strip off the ligamentum plantare longum, which extends between the os calcis and the cuboid. This ligament is often contracted and, if so, produces a concavity of the foot at the outer border. By keeping close to the bone in stripping, one is at a safe distance from the plantar vessels and

nerves. When the stripping has been completed, correction of
the foot is accomplished by wrenching and in more severe cases
by such bone operations as it may be necessary to add, according
to the degree of the skeletal deformities.

The subcutaneous and skin layers are closed by layers and the
foot is put up in plaster in extreme dorsiflexion. At the end of ten
days or two weeks, the cast is removed, the skin sutures taken out,

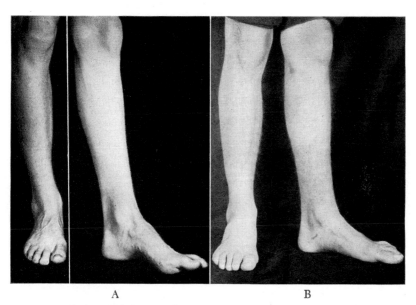

A   B

FIG. 88. A high-arched foot. A, before operation; B, after a midtarsal-arthrodesis
operation.

and a new cast applied with the foot in the position of maximum
correction. If no operation has been performed on the bones, the
cast may be removed in two weeks and a properly balanced shoe
supplied. It is usually advisable to place a support under the forepart of the foot for a time, or to place a metatarsal bar in the shoe
to raise the metatarsal heads and thus continue the correction
as the foot is used.

MIDTARSAL ARTHRODESIS. Occasionally a cavus foot is encountered in which the arch is so high, the ball of the foot so prominent, and the contracture of the toes so extreme, that elongation

of the plantar fascia alone will be insufficient to correct deformity. When this condition is encountered, a wedge osteotomy of the tarsus may be properly performed. A wedge of bone, base upward, is removed from the navicular cuneiform joint and from the body of the cuboid bone, sufficient to reduce the elevated or cavus arch to a satisfactory height. This type of operation does not interfere with lateral motion of the foot, and the results are, as a rule, very satisfactory (Fig. 88).

SUMMARY

The importance of correcting faulty foot balance in the adolescent period cannot be overemphasized if future trouble is to be avoided, and such correction should be insisted upon even to the extent of advising operative correction if necessary. There are many, qualified to hold an opinion, who do not believe that operative treatment has any place in the management of foot imbalance in the adolescent period or in any period. To those who hold such views the proposal to correct foot imbalance by operation, when necessary, will not find acceptance; however, our experience has convinced us of the soundness of using intelligently planned operative measures for the correction of fundamental faults in the unbalanced foot of adolescence in properly selected cases, and we believe that this position is being more widely accepted each year.

9

FOOT IMBALANCE IN THE ADULT

Functional foot disorders, the result of foot imbalance, and deformities which persistent imbalance produce, are among the common incapacitating conditions which affect the human race. Foot imbalance, then, must be ranked as an important health condition which vitally affects the well-being and efficiency of a very considerable number of people. For this reason, it is deserving of thoughtful consideration and study by the medical profession. Notwithstanding the importance of foot disorders as an economic problem, few in the profession outside the orthopedic specialty have any understanding of the common disorders of the foot with respect to symptomatology, diagnosis, and treatment; moreover, most physicians and surgeons, and indeed not a few orthopedic surgeons feel that it is beneath their dignity to treat functional foot disorders. This attitude has been largely responsible for the general belief that the care of the disabling foot conditions does not lie within the medical field. Whitman has said, "If one has a cut or a felon on his finger, he goes to the hospital and is treated by a surgeon; if the foot is painful, he is the subject of ridicule." Whitman might well have added that if a physician is consulted, the patient will, in all probability, be sent to a shoe store for treatment. As the result of the indifference which the medical profession has displayed toward the treatment of symptom-producing foot conditions, their management has fallen largely into extraprofessional hands, shoe salesmen, manufacturers of arch supports of various kinds, and irregular practitioners, to the detriment of the patient and loss of prestige for the attending physician. Since foot imbalance is almost as great a scourge to humanity as arthritis, it is difficult to explain why this position should be taken by the profession, unless it is that, like arthritis, foot disabilities do not shorten life and are not contagious in origin and so fail to arouse professional interest. Yet it cannot be denied that foot imbalance is a problem of great

sociologic and economic importance and should be of deep interest
to all practicing physicians.

It is not difficult for a physician to acquire sufficient knowledge
of foot balance to enable him to diagnose the presence of imbalance and suggest treatment, or, at least, to insist that competent
advice be sought. Treatment of the simple and uncomplicated
case is well within the capacity of the practitioner who is willing
to give the subject some study; the management of the more
severe forms, however, usually requires an experience and arma-
mentarium which he does not possess and necessitates the attention of one specially trained in their correction. It would
seem, then, since foot disability is a condition for which advice
is constantly being sought, that it would be well worthwhile for
the profession to acquire at least a working knowledge of foot
disorders and their causes so that intelligent advice could be given
when occasion arises.

Functional foot disorders do not begin at the time of the onset
of symptoms; these simply indicate the breakdown of a structure
which has long been functioning at a mechanical disadvantage.
Certainly it seems difficult to conceive that a normal foot could
become suddenly insufficient except from extraordinary strain or
under the burden of an enormously increased load—occurrences
which are not common. The only logical conclusion, then, is
that functional foot disorders in the adult must, in the majority
of instances, be looked upon as the culmination of years of use
under adverse conditions—conditions which had their inception
in early life. Faults in the architecture of the foot of congenital
origin are certainly active in producing faulty foot attitude from
the time the first steps are taken. Faults in architecture which
result from distorting stresses and strains must have their be-
ginnings in the developmental period, that is, in childhood. It
seems, then, that in seeking for the explanation of foot imbalance
in the adult, we should, in the majority of cases, look for evidence
of long-standing faulty architecture owing to congenital faults
or the result of distorting stresses. On the other hand, it must be
admitted that there are conditions of life which throw an unusual
strain upon the foot and which may eventually cause even a normal

foot to break down and become symptom-producing. That systemic disease, occupation, and living conditions play a very important role as a contributing cause of symptom-producing foot conditions is unquestioned. It is consistently reported that functional foot disorders do not exist among races which do not wear shoes, while their prevalence among the so-called civilized races is well known. Civilization has imposed upon the workers long hours of labor in the standing position with little relief from weight-bearing; has replaced resilient earth with level pavements and floors, constructed of nonresilient materials; has encased the feet in footwear which too often is poorly designed and incorrectly fitted. These conditions plus the economic drive for existence or advancement which requires strenuous, sustained effort and wears down and debilitates the individual generally, unquestionably make heavy demands upon the foot of normal design and construction and must eventually result in the breaking down of the foot of limited capacity. Functional foot disorders, then, are due in the main to structural defects and excessive work; or, stated in another way, to lowered capacity of the foot to meet the excessive demands made upon it by occupation and environment.

TYPES OF FOOT IMBALANCE

In the foot of childhood we have one basic type of foot imbalance—pes planus; in the adolescent type we have two basic types—pes planus, pes cavus. In the adult foot, we have three basic types of imbalance. They are:

1. Depression of the longitudinal arch, pes planus or flatfoot (Fig. 89).
2. Elevation of the longitudinal arch, or pes cavus (Fig. 90).
3. Depression of the anterior or metatarsal arch (Fig. 91).

This third type of foot imbalance may be questioned as being a separate entity, for it seldom occurs unaccompanied by some fault in the longitudinal arch (pes planus or pes cavus) granted that at times such faults may be extremely slight. However, in its most serious form, the symptoms of depression of the metatarsal arch overshadow those due to faults in the longitudinal arch, and it seems best to consider foot imbalance in the adult under the three headings listed above.

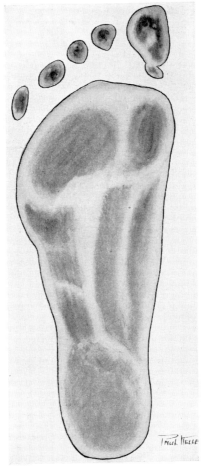

Fig. 89. Pedograph of a foot in weight-bearing with depression of the longitudinal arch, pes planus or flatfoot.

Pes Planus (Flatfoot)

By a flatfoot is meant one in which there is inrolling or pronation of the foot and a depression or lowering of the longitudinal arch.

ETIOLOGY

The following are the most common causes of pes planus or flatfoot:

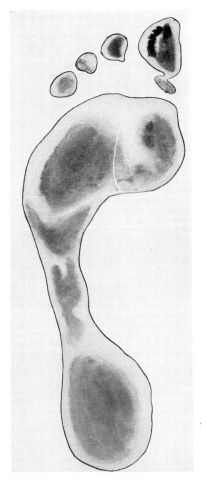

FIG. 90. Pedograph of a foot in weight-bearing with a high longitudinal arch, pes cavus.

1. **Congenital deformities or abnormalities of the bones of the foot,** such as short metatarsal I, metatarsus varus primus, hypermobility of the first metatarsal segment, and accessory

scaphoid, or prehallux. These congenital abnormalities are in reality throwbacks to the arboreal foot, as has been clearly demonstrated by Morton. Their effect is to decrease the stability of the anterior pillar of the inner longitudinal arch of the foot (the first

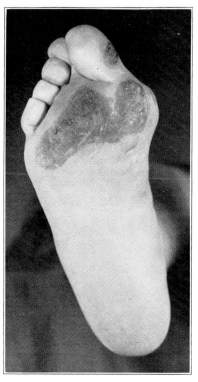

Fig. 91. Depression of the anterior or metatarsal arch.

metatarsal head), and so permit inrolling or pronation of the foot and eventually descent of the longitudinal arch (Figs. 92-93).

2. **Acquired deformities of the foot,** such as hallux valgus and disturbances in the foot architecture due to fractures of the foot bones and loss of toes or other parts of the foot. Hallux valgus, by depriving the medial side of the foot of the supporting action of the great toe, allows the foot to roll in, or pronate, and favors the descent of the longitudinal arch (Fig. 94). Fractures of the

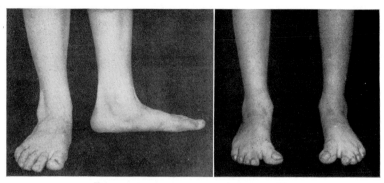

FIG. 92   FIG. 93

FIG. 92. Depression of the longitudinal arch and pronation with a short first
metatarsal.
FIG. 93. Pronating weak foot with a short and deformed metatarsal I.

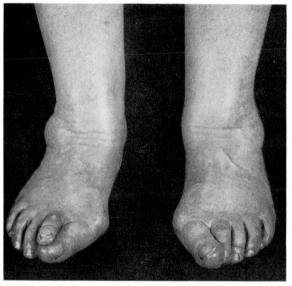

FIG. 94. Hallux valgus allows the foot to roll in or pronate and favors descent of
the longitudinal arch.

foot bones, particularly of the os calcis, frequently result in depression of the longitudinal arch, through changes brought about in the relations of the bones of the foot to each other.

3. **Short heel cord.** A short heel tendon produces deforming stresses within the adult foot just as it does in the growing and adolescent foot. (1) As a short heel cord does not permit complete

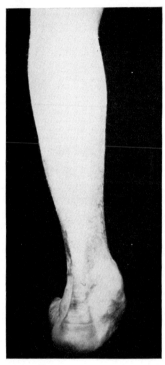

FIG. 95. Pes planus with marked pronation owing to a contracted heel tendon which is seen displaced laterally.

dorsoflexion of the foot, it throws the burden of weight-bearing largely upon the anterior part of the foot. In walking, this concentration of weight on the forepart of the foot causes downward and inward displacement of the subastragalar joint, and in time descent of the longitudinal arch. (2) The pull which a short heel cord exerts on the os calcis tends to roll it inward and tilt the subastragalar joint downward and inward and to depress the longitudinal arch of the foot (Fig. 95).

4. **Weakness or deficiency of the leg and foot muscles.** Muscle deficiency may be true muscle weakness owing to debility caused by illness or the result of actual muscle paralysis, as for

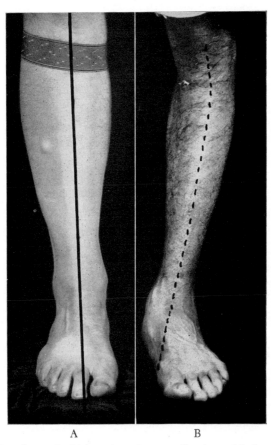

A   B

FIG. 96. Bow leg and tibial torsion. A, normally the weight-bearing line falls between the first and second metatarsal; B, with tibial torsion the weight bearing line falls medial to metatarsal I.

example, infantile paralysis. Muscle deficiency may be relative; that is, not due to actual weakness of the muscles but to the fact that they are incapable of performing the work required of them, as when superimposed weight is excessive. Muscle weakness causes flatfoot largely through the inability of the muscles to maintain the leg in an approximately vertical plane over the foot.

When the supinators are insufficient, the foot rolls inward at the subastragalar joint, there is concentration of weight over the medial side of the foot, and the longitudinal arch, under the stress of faulty weight-bearing, descends.

5. **Improper footwear.** There can be no doubt that wearing extremely high-heeled shoes and shoes which are short or of an improper width plays a part in the causation of foot imbalance. Improper shoes are chiefly harmful in that they throw the foot out of balance and interfere with reasonable freedom of movement by crowding the toes and the forepart of the foot. Under such conditions the foot cannot function properly and any weakness present will be accentuated, and even a normal foot may eventually break down.

6. **Knock knee, bow leg, and tibial torsion.** Knock knee, bow leg, and tibial torsion cause a shift in the line of transmitted weight so that the weight stresses fall upon the foot in an abnormal manner. The line of transmitted weight normally passes approximately through the middle of the patella and falls between metatarsals I and II. With knock knee, because the line of the tibia angulates outward, the line of weight-bearing falls through metatarsal I or medial to it. With bow leg and tibial torsion, because the line of the tibia angulates out and then in, the line of weight-bearing falls through metatarsal I or medial to it, just as it does in knock knee, and the weight-bearing thrust is on the medial side of the foot (Fig. 96). In both instances there is a concentration of weight stresses on the medial side of the foot which rolls downward and inward at the subastragalar joint with eventual depression of the longitudinal arch.

PATHOLOGY

The pathology in pes planus consists of changes in the architecture and structure of the foot, the result of disturbance of its normal balance.

The foot is held in balance on the leg in two planes: The lateral plane and the anterior-posterior plane. In pes planus, the chief disturbance in balance is in the lateral plane. Normally, the line of transmitted weight passes through the middle of the patella and falls between metatarsals I and II. When, for any cause, the line of transmitted weight falls through metatarsal I or medial to it, there is a concentration of weight on the inner side of the foot, which rolls downward and inward at the subastragalar joint, the longitudinal arch is lowered or depressed, and the foot assumes the position of pronation. Continued use of the foot in

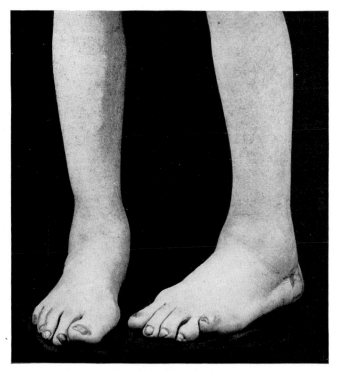

Fig. 97. Rigid pes planus with pronation.

such a position of strain brings about a gradual stretching of the ligaments, displacement, or at least loss, of the normal compact arrangement of the foot bones, and finally tiring and weakening of the supporting muscles on the medial side of the foot and shortening of the muscles on the lateral side of the foot. Such a foot is relaxed and weak and decidedly subnormal in its ability to bear weight and to meet the demands of locomotion. Such a foot, however, can always be brought into a position of balance manually. If the causes responsible for pes planus continue active over a long period of time, prolonged irritation of the ligaments and joints of the foot may result in proliferative changes in these ligaments and joints, particularly if an arthritic diathesis is present. Whether a true arthritis develops or the changes in the foot joints are merely those of chronic irritation, the range of motion in these joints is reduced or even lost, and the foot becomes fixed in the position of deformity and a rigid pes planus results. With the foot fixed rigidly in pronation and eversion, the peroneal muscles contract and shorten, and so contribute to the rigidity of the foot, and provide an additional check to joint movement (Fig. 97). Such a rigid pes planus is much more serious than the relaxed type, since the rigidity of the foot does not permit manual correction, and restoration of normal alignment can be brought about only by forcible manipulation.

In addition to the changes in the bones, ligaments, and muscles of the foot and leg, other soft parts, such as the blood vessels and nerves supplying the foot may be interfered with. Interference with the blood supply may result in venous congestion and swelling of the foot and ankle. Interference with the nerve supply may cause pain, hyperesthesia, and paresthesia in the various parts of the foot.

SYMPTOMS

The symptoms of pes planus are those which might be expected from the pathology present and are both subjective and objective.

Subjective

1. **Pain and discomfort** are the most outstanding complaints in pes planus. In the beginning, the term "discomfort" probably describes the situation more accurately than "pain," since a "tired feeling" in the longitudinal arch and the calves of the legs is often the first indication of foot strain. This "tired feeling" gradually increases in intensity and in time becomes real, and often disabling, pain. When the painful stage is reached, the discomfort usually becomes localized in the region of the scaphoid bone and the subastragalar joint but may include the entire foot.

Cramping pain in the calf of the leg is not infrequently an outstanding subjective symptom. This condition is due to muscle strain and tire.

2. **General tire and lack of endurance** is a frequent complaint. Such general tiring is due to the increased effort required for normal activity, because of lack of spring and resiliency in the foot, and muscle tire.

3. **Knee pain** is occasionally complained of. Such knee pain is caused by abnormal strain brought upon the internal lateral ligament of the knee joint through the shifting inward of the line of transmitted weight owing to the disturbed relationship between the foot and the leg (pronation).

4. **Backache.** Pain in the lower back radiating into the lateral aspect of the thigh is an even more common complaint than the knee pain. The downward tilting of the front of the pelvis and the upward and forward tilting of the back of the pelvis, which results from inrolling of the feet, produces a hollow back. The faulty posture which results throws an increased strain on the lumbar muscles and ligaments and is responsible for the backache in pes planus.

5. **At times excessive perspiring** of the feet is complained of.

Objective

When making an examination for objective evidence of pes planus or flatfoot, the position assumed by the patient should be that already described in the chapter on "Examination." The position taken is, standing with the feet parallel and about three inches apart, the patient first facing the examiner and then facing away from the examiner. When the examination in a standing position is completed, the foot should be re-examined in the sitting position.

With the patient standing, the following evidence of an unbalanced foot indicates a pes planus or flatfoot (Fig. 98).

Depression of the longitudinal arch. This may be comparatively slight or may be quite extreme in degree. In the latter case, there will be practically no arch observable.

Pronation or inrolling of the foot so that the line of transmitted weight falls through metatarsal I or even medial to the inner border of the foot.

Prominence of the scaphoid bone owing to pronation or downward and inward rolling of the subastragalar joint, and prominence of the internal malleolus owing to eversion of the foot.

Abnormalities of the first metatarsal segment: Shortness of metatarsal I is suggested by shortness of the great toe compared

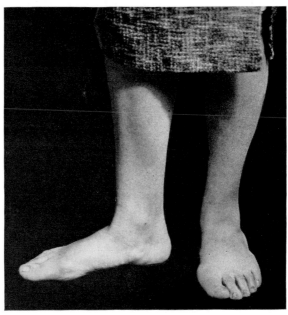

FIG. 98. Pes planus or flatfoot. Depression of the longitudinal arch, inrolling or pronation, prominence of the scaphoid, and mild hallux valgus.

with the second and other toes (see Fig. 92). Prominence of the great toe with lateral projection of the great toe (hallux valgus) and a broad, splayed out forefoot indicate a metatarsus varus primus (see Figs. 93-94).

With the patient sitting, inspection of the foot will usually present additional evidences of abnormality, such as:

A flattening out or undue prominence of the ball of the foot if the anterior or metatarsal arch is involved. Tenderness to palpation is usually present in the region of the scaphoid bone and the head of the astragalus and over the plantar surface of the middle cuneiform bone (Fig. 99). The tenderness at these points is probably due to synovitis of the important joints in these locations. The presence of a short heel cord is indicated by lessening of the range of dorsal flexion in the foot with the knee extended

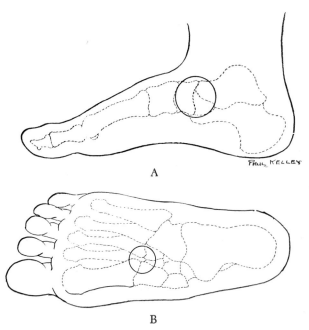

A

B

FIG. 99. Points of tenderness in foot imbalance: A, over the astragaloscaphoid joint; B, tenderness to palpation is usually present on the sole of the foot under the cuneiform second metatarsal joint.

and the foot held in mild adduction; the adducted male foot should dorsally flex to 85 or 90 degrees; the female foot to about 90 degrees. An abnormal range of dorsiflexion of the first metatarsal bone indicates that a hypermobile first metatarsal segment is present. Callosities under the heads of metatarsals I, II and V, and at times over the entire ball of the foot are frequently observed.

In the rigid type of flatfoot, the tendons of the peroneus longus

and brevis will be short and contracted, the lateral mobility of
the foot will be seriously limited, and it will be impossible to
bring the foot into a position of correction.

X-ray examination of a symptom-producing foot should be
made if possible and should be insisted upon if a short first metatarsal, metatarsus varus primus, or any other structural abnor-

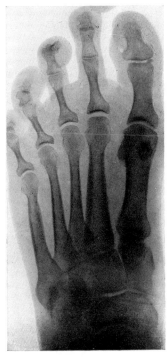

FIG. 100. Dorsiplantar x-ray of a foot showing a short metatarsal I and overdevelop
ment of metatarsal II.

mality is suspected. The most important information derived from
an x-ray is whether a short first metatarsal with overdevelopment
of the second metatarsal, a metatarsus varus primus with wide
separation between metatarsals I and II, a hypermobile first
metatarsal segment, or arthritic changes in the foot joints are
present (Fig. 100). The plate should be a dorsiplantar view made
with the patient standing.

The diagnosis of pes planus is based upon subjective symptoms, objective findings, and x-ray evidence. Subjective symptoms may be summarized as pain, discomfort, and tiring of the foot; associated with these local symptoms, we have knee pain or backache in a definite percentage of cases. It is the information supplied by physical examination of the foot which must be relied upon to determine the type of foot imbalance which is present in any given case, and the importance of a careful examination of the symptom-producing foot cannot be overemphasized.

As part of the diagnosis, the evaluation of the part played by structural defects in the weight-bearing bones, such as shortness of metatarsal I, hypermobile first metatarsal segment, metatarsus varus primus, and accessory scaphoid, and faulty weight-bearing stresses owing to short heel cord, knock knee, bow leg, and tibial torsion is important. Such conditions if present are, in all probability, the primary cause of the functional foot disorder, and their correction or at least their amelioration as far as possible will constitute a very important part of the plan of management determined upon.

X-ray examination plays a very important part in arriving at a diagnosis, as it yields definite information as to the presence or absence of structural defects or deficiencies in the architecture of the foot. If the x-ray is not utilized in diagnosis, information necessary to effective treatment may be missed.

TREATMENT

In pes planus, we have a foot characterized by inrolling or pronation, displacement of the line of transmitted weight toward the medial side of the foot, depression of the longitudinal arch, and tired and often spastic muscles. The problem in treatment presented is then three-fold: (1) To correct the pronation of the foot and bring the line of transmitted weight toward the lateral side of the foot, so that there may be a proper distribution of the weight stresses over the entire foot; (2) to elevate and support the depressed longitudinal arch, and thereby reduce strain on the stretched plantar ligaments and allow them to shorten and hold the bones of the foot in the compact arrangement necessary if normal architecture, or at least an architecture which will insure reasonable efficiency, is to be maintained; (3) to build up the natural supports of the arches, the muscles and ligaments, so that they may function as effectively as possible and maintain the foot in a position of balance.

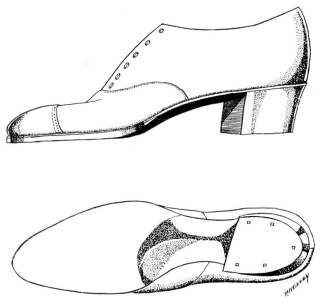

FIG. 101. Proper type of oxford for women. Side view shows cut of upper and height of heel. Lower view shows cut of sole with ample toe room; heel extended slightly forward on the inner side to give added support to the shank.

The first two of these desiderata, the proper distribution of weight stresses and elevation of the longitudinal arch, are secured by bringing the foot into balance or as near balance as possible. An unbalanced foot is brought into balance by wearing a shoe of the proper type, balanced to meet the requirements of the foot to be treated, and using an arch support in conjunction with such a balanced shoe. The third, strengthening of the muscles and ligaments, is brought about by relieving these structures from strain; this is accomplished by correction of faulty foot attitude, and by the use of exercises and physiotherapy to build up muscle strength and ligamentous tone.

Shoes. The subject of footwear is discussed in chapter 10 and you are referred to that chapter for detailed information; here the features of a correct shoe, which are in our opinion important, will merely be enumerated (Fig. 101). They are:

1. The shoe should be of the oxford type. A Bal or Blucher design may be used.
2. The lines should be straight on the inner side and the outer side should not curve in too acutely but should taper gradually to a moderately pointed toe.
3. There must be ample room in the ball of the shoe for free action of the forepart of the foot and toes.
4. The sole should be the flat type and sufficiently heavy to give support.
5. The heel should be of the straight-side type. For men, the height of the heel should be six- to seventh-eighths of an inch; for women, twelve-eighths to fourteen-eighths.
6. The shank should be moderately broad and should be given rigidity by having incorporated into it a steel shank extending from the heel to the bend of the toe at the ball.
7. The counter should fit the heel snugly and the vamp should lace rather firmly over the instep.
8. The shoe should be long enough to extend a finger's breadth beyond the tip of the great toe.

A shoe of this type should be worn most of the time and always during the hours of the day when the foot is being subjected to the strain of greatest use. If a shoe of the correct type is worn during what may be termed "the working hours of the day," it may be replaced by one of lighter weight and more pleasing design for evening wear and for dress occasions. The selection of the correct shoe for men is usually not difficult, as most men's shoes are sensible in design and fulfill most of the qualifications listed above. Conventional types of women's shoes are, as a rule, of high-heeled, pointed-toe design with a narrow shank, and thin turned soles, a type of footwear which is unsuited to a foot with any symptomatic disorder. Suggestions for change from this type of shoe to one of oxford design with a reasonably high heel usually meet with considerable resistance, but if results are to be obtained, it is necessary that a firm stand be taken, and the wearing of a well-designed supporting type of shoe be insisted upon, at least until symptoms are relieved. With the disappearance of acute symptoms, greater latitude in selection of footwear may be permitted. Usually, however, if the foot has been made comfortable, it requires little persuasion to have the patient continue to use a correct shoe for general wear.

Supports. There is probably no single therapeutic measure in medicine about which more diversity of opinion is held than upon the kind of support which should be used in the treatment of static faults in the foot. Whatever the difference of opinion may be as to the best type of support, it is generally conceded that some device which will support the arch is necessary for the successful management of a foot which is unbalanced and causing symptoms, the type of support being a matter of personal preference and experience. Broadly speaking, arch supports may be divided into: (1) rigid supports, made of metal, celluloid, or composition; and (2) nonrigid supports made of leather, hard felt, or sponge rubber.

RIGID SUPPORTS. The Whitman foot plate is generally conceded to be the best form of rigid support yet devised, and it is the one usually prescribed. Properly made and fitted, it is most efficient and gives effective service.

WHITMAN FOOT PLATE. Properly to construct a Whitman foot plate, it must be modeled upon an exact cast of the foot to be treated. The cast is made in the following manner: The patient is seated in a chair opposite another chair, somewhat lower in height, on which is laid a thick pad of cotton covered with a square of cotton cloth. Plaster of Paris is then added to water until a mixture of the consistency of thick cream is obtained. The patient's knee is now flexed and the outer side of the foot, previously rubbed with talcum powder, is allowed to sink into the plaster which has been poured upon the cloth. The foot should be slightly plantar-flexed with its transverse measurement perpen-

dicular to the chair. It is an advantage to lift the foot and have
the surface of the second chair so inclined that its highest side
is toward the front of the foot. This, together with the weight
of the limb, will cause the foot to assume a position of slight
adduction. The borders of the cloth are raised and the plaster
is pressed against the foot until rather more than half is covered.
As soon as the plaster is hard, it is removed, its surface covered

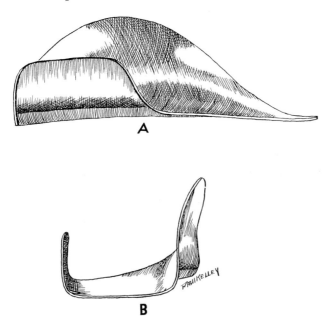

FIG. 102. Whitman foot plate. A, side view; B, rear view.

with vaseline, and it is temporarily replaced on the foot. The re-
mainder of the foot is then covered with plaster. The two halves
are then removed, again greased, and bandaged together. The
interior is dampened with soapsuds, then filled with plaster cream.
On removing the shell, a cast of the foot is secured which, when
properly made, should stand upright without inclination to one
side or the other.

In most instances, it is an advantage to deepen the model at
the inner and outer segments of the arch, in order that the arches
of the brace may be slightly exaggerated, especially at the heel,

so that depression of the anterior extremity of the os calcis may be prevented. If the outer border of the cast is flattened by pressure, a little plaster should be added to approximate it to its normal contour. If there is prominence of the scaphoid or the head of the astragalus on the inner side, the cast should be thickened in the model over these parts so that there is very slight, if any, pressure upon them when the brace is completed.

The brace is outlined on the model. The material to be used is eighteen- to twenty-gauge steel. The brace consists of three parts (Fig. 102): (1) the main part of the brace, fitted to the sole, extends from the center of the heel to a point just behind the ball of the great toe; it offers no restraint to the normal motions of the foot; (2) a broad internal upright portion which covers and protects the astragaloscaphoid joint, rising above the scaphoid bone; (3) an external upright arm which covers the calcaneocuboid joint and holds the foot securely in place on the brace.

Once the brace has been constructed as described, it must be carefully adjusted to meet the needs of the foot of the individual. Alterations in the foot plate are made by hammering it with a round-headed hammer on a lead anvil; by gentle and properly placed blows, the plate can be moulded so that there will be no impingement of the brace on any bony prominence. It may require several attempts to align the foot plate so that it is entirely comfortable.

NONRIGID SUPPORTS. Nonrigid supports have, the authors believe, certain advantages over the rigid form, and they have for years used this type in the treatment of foot imbalance in children, adolescents, and adults. The advantages of nonrigid supports are two-fold: First, they are easier to make, fit, and alter; and second, they are much more resilient than supports made of metal or celluloid, provide a softer and more comfortable support to the arch, and interfere less with the action of the foot than do the rigid type. A nonrigid support, however, requires a more rigid and carefully balanced shoe than does the rigid support, as the shoe must supply a firm foundation upon which the support may rest. There are a number of different materials from which nonrigid supports can be fashioned, but piano felt and sponge rubber are those most generally used. The authors have for years used a non-rigid support made of sponge rubber with uniformly good results. As this support has proved very satisfactory, and is not difficult to adjust, it will be described in some detail for the benefit of those who may wish to employ it in the treatment of painful foot disorders.

AUTHORS' NONRIGID SUPPORTS. The support is made of sponge rubber of fairly firm consistency. It has been found most satis-

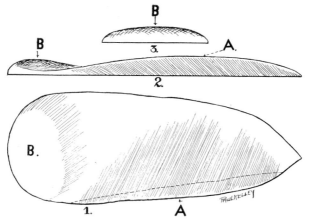

FIG. 103. Stock sponge-rubber support. A, longitudinal arch portion; B, transverse arch portion. 1, shape of inlay; 2, contour of support (lateral view); 3, contour of transverse arch section of support.

factory to have the support manufactured in the rough by a rubber manufacturing company, as it can be fabricated in bulk at a very low cost. Supports or inlays should be made in three sizes: Small, medium, and large; with these sizes practically any foot can be fitted.

The support has two parts (Fig. 103): A longitudinal section for the longitudinal arch, and an anterior section for the metatarsal arch; as the support is designed to elevate both the longitudinal arch and the metatarsal or transverse arch, these two sections are necessary. The longitudinal portion of the support (Fig. 103A) is approximately one-fourth of an inch thick on the inner side at its highest point and tapers to a feather edge on the outer side and posteriorly. Anteriorly on its inner side, it is bevelled somewhat and gradually merges with the anterior elevation for the metatarsal arch. The anterior section of the support (Fig. 103B) is rounded in shape to conform approxi-

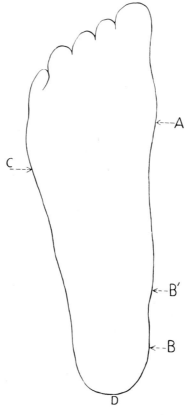

Fig. 104. Outline of sole of foot with measurements for the support. A, position of first metatarsal head; B′, position of sustentaculum tali; C, position of fifth metatarsal head. The distance from A to B is the length of the support. The distance from A to D is the distance of the anterior margin of the support from the back of the shoe.

mately to the outline of the heads of the metatarsal bones; the height at its anterior margin is from three-sixteenths to one-fourth of an inch. A sponge-rubber support of this type may be readily adapted to the requirements of the foot, as it can be fashioned to give any desired height to the longitudinal or anterior sections, limited only by the original height of the support.

Fitting and shaping the support is not a haphazard procedure, but, on the contrary, requires reasonable care and accuracy. To determine the proper length of the support, an outline of the foot should be made or a pedigraph taken; on the inner side of this outline, the position of the heads of metatarsals I and II,

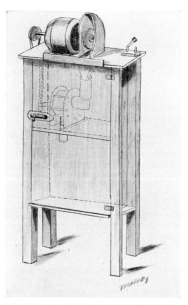

Fɪɢ. 105. Motor-driven emery wheel used to smooth and skive the rubber supports. Suction apparatus below to care for rubber dust.

and the position of the anterior border of the os calcis should be marked (Fig. 104). On the outer side the position of the head of metatarsal V should be marked. The support should extend from just posterior to the head of the second metatarsal bone to well back under the heel; its highest point should lie under the anterior one-third of the os calcis (sustentaculum tali) Fig. 104B'. The width of the anterior part of the support should be the distance from the lateral side of the head of metatarsal I to the medial side of the head of metatarsal V. With a little experience, the outline or pedigraph may be dispensed with and the support fitted directly to the sole, using the landmarks already described.

After a support of the proper width and length has been selected, it is fashioned to give the exact shape desired and the amount of elevation determined upon as necessary to support the anterior and longitudinal arches. One of the advantages of

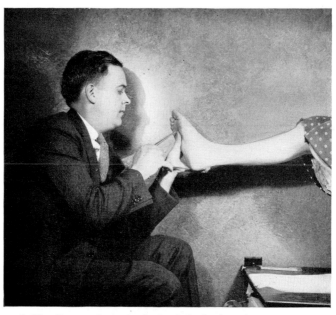

FIG. 106. The distance from the back of the heel to the posterior aspect of the second metatarsal head is taken with a caliper and represents the distance from the anterior margin of the inlay to the rear of the insole. This measurement is used for the placement of the inlay in the shoe.

this type of support is the latitude which it allows in shaping and elevation. Alterations in the height and shape of the original molded support may be made with a sharp knife, but they are more readily and conveniently effected by grinding on a small, coarse, emery wheel (Fig. 105). The use of an emery wheel makes it possible to shape the support smoothly and evenly in a few moments and converts what seems to be a rather complicated, laborious and time-consuming procedure into quite a simple one.

When the support has been fitted and fashioned into the desired form, it is placed in the shoe and firmly fastened to the

insole. If the support is to be comfortable and efficient, it must
be placed in the shoe in correct relation to the longitudinal and
metatarsal arches; in order that this may be accomplished, it is

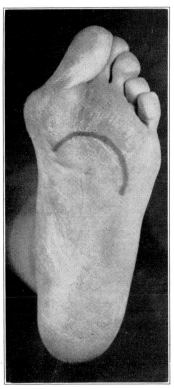

FIG. 107. The impression of the anterior margin of the support on the sole of the
foot is a guide for proper adjustment of the support.

desirable to use some method of determining accurately its proper
position in the shoe. The exact position of the support is determined by measuring the distance from the head of metatarsal
II to the back of the heel with a caliper (Fig. 106). This caliper
distance is used to locate the inlay by placing one point of the
caliper flush with the counter of the heel when the other caliper
point will indicate the head of metatarsal II and, therefore, the
position of the anterior end of the support. Occasionally, usually
because of some peculiarity of the foot, this measurement will

not be exactly correct, and it is always desirable to have the patient walk about for a few moments with the supports in place to get an impression of the support on the sole of the foot. The shoe should then be removed and the position of the support checked by the impression made (Fig. 107). By making an out-

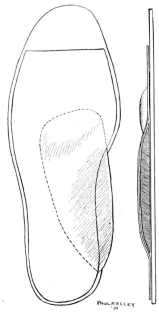

FIG. 108. The support is covered with leather or leather substitute.

line drawing of the support on the history and marking down the caliper distance from the heel to the head of the second metatarsal on the drawing, it is possible to place a support in a number of shoes without requiring the presence of the patient.

In fastening the support in the shoe, it is best to use two or three shoe tacks. Large headed carpet tacks should not be used. After being placed in position, the support should be covered by thin leather or leather substitute, both of which can be obtained from shoe supply houses at a small cost (Fig. 108).

In designing or making any form of arch support, rigid or non-rigid, it is important to keep in mind several basic facts. In pes planus our aim is to correct inrolling or pronation and to elevate the depressed longitudinal arch and the metatarsal arch when it is depressed. Since inrolling of the foot or pronation of the foot is the precursor of descent of the longitudinal and metatarsal arches with resultant muscle and ligamentous strain, correction

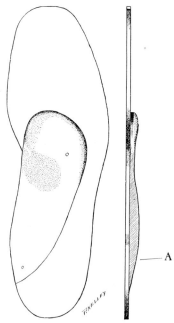

FIG. 109. Shape, contour and placement of the support for pes planus or flatfoot
A indicates high point of support.

of pronation is the keystone of treatment of pes planus. Pronation can be prevented only by maintaining the os calcis in a varus position. The os calcis can be held in a varus position only by elevation and outward tilting or rolling or the anterior part of the os calcis, while at the same time the heel is prevented from sliding outward in the shoe. As the os calcis rolls outward, it rotates the subastragalar joint upward and outward, elevates the head of the astragalus, the scaphoid and cuneiform bones, and locks the calcaneocuboid joint firmly. This corrects pronation and increases the height of the longitudinal arch. To roll the os calcis outward, it is necessary that the support be high enough under the anterior part of the os calcis to exert a direct upward thrust against the sustentaculum tali. The high point of support on the inner side should then be well back under the sustentaculum tali; the support should continue forward at about the same height to the scaphoid bone, from which point it slopes downward and forward rather acutely (Fig. 109). Posteriorly, the support should bevel down rather acutely from the high point, but it should extend well back under the heel. A support so shaped uses the natural mechanics of the foot to correct pronation and elevate the longitudinal arch by assisting the bones of the foot to assume their normal relationship to each other, so that they become a compact, comparatively non-yielding framework. If the high point of the support is placed under the scaphoid and the head of the astragalus, it can act only as a jack to force the arch upward; this is an almost impossible task against the burden of the superimposed weight and is mechanically unsound. The thickness of the support at its highest point is determined by the amount of thrust against the sustentaculum tali required to overcome pronation. It is obvious that the height of the support must be limited to an elevation which the foot will tolerate comfortably.

The anterior section of the support should be skived or bevelled on the inner side so that the elevation begins at the lateral side of the head of metatarsal I. It should be bevelled slightly on its outer side so that the elevation ends on the medial side of metatarsal V. The height of the anterior extremity of the anterior section is determined by the amount of elevation of the metatarsal arch which seems necessary. When hallux valgus is present, the inner side of the anterior section of the inlay is bevelled off rather acutely, and that part of the longitudinal section which lies under the first metatarsal bone should be skived down to a greater extent than in the ordinary support, in order to prevent undue pressure against the enlarged and sensitive great toe joint.

It is advisable when determining the height of the support or inlay to be used to avoid making it too high at the start of treatment, as this may cause unnecessary discomfort. It is best to use a reasonable elevation at first and gradually increase the height as the foot acquires tolerance to the support. The height of both portions of the support may be increased from time to time by placing shaped pieces of hard piano felt or sponge rubber under the support, between it and the insole of the shoe (Fig. 110).

Platforms. Dudley Morton has called attention to the part played by a short metatarsal I with concentration of weight upon metatarsal II in causing disturbance of foot balance. To retransfer to metatarsal I the weight which it should normally bear, Morton advised that a platform be placed under the head of the short first metatarsal bone and in this way raise the supporting surface beneath it to a level where the desired amount of contact between

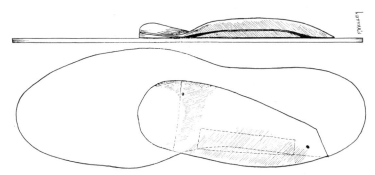

Fig. 110. Method of raising the longitudinal or transverse arch portion of the support by the addition of thin wedges of felt or sponge rubber.

the first metatarsal head and the bearing surface is gained. In other words, the shortness of the first metatarsal bone is compensated for by raising the bearing surface under its head. Following Morton's suggestion, we have used such a platform with definite improvement in foot balance in a number of cases (Fig. 111). Experience has convinced the authors, however, that a platform alone is not sufficient to relieve symptoms in cases showing a short first metatarsal in which definite pronation is present; it has been necessary in such cases to use both a platform and a support under the longitudinal arch. Such a combination has proved very satisfactory in properly selected cases. The platform used is fashioned from sponge rubber; it is from one-eighth to three-sixteenths of an inch in thickness and is shaped to fit the lines of the inner border of the shoe. The regular support must

be skived down anteriorly on its inner margin sufficiently to allow
room for the added bulk of the platform when it is used (Fig. 112).

Shoe Alterations. A correctly designed shoe and properly made
arch support in some instances fail to bring the unbalanced foot
into a balanced position. When this situation arises, alterations
in the shoe which change its balance may be utilized further to

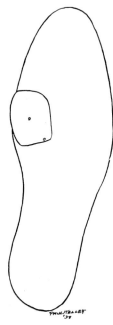

Fɪɢ. 111. Metatarsal platform placed in the shoe and used to elevate the head
of metatarsal I.

improve the position of the foot. Three alterations in the sole
and heel of the shoe have proved useful in the authors' experience:
A metatarsal wedge, elevation or the heel of the shoe on the inner
side, and an extended or Thomas heel.

A metatarsal wedge is a wedge of leather one-eighth to three-
sixteenths of an inch thick and approximately an inch and a half
long placed between the layers of the sole of the shoe on the
outer side; its high point should lie just beneath the head of the
fifth metatarsal bone (Fig. 113). If this wedge is too long or is

placed too far forward, it tends to turn the outer side of the sole up and press upon the fifth toe and cause discomfort. Such a

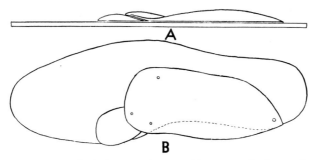

FIG. 112. First metatarsal platform used in combination with the regular support. A, side view; B, placement in the shoe.

metatarsal wedge prevents supinatory torsion of the forepart of the foot and enhances the efficiency of the support under the

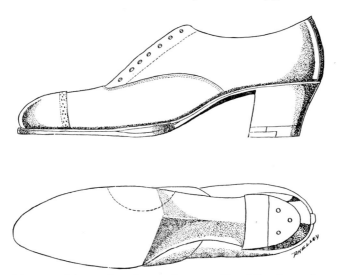

FIG. 113. Metatarsal wedge on the outer side of the shoe sole.

longitudinal arch. It also decreases the tendency of the foot to slide toward the outer side of the shoe and off the support; this outward sliding of the foot decreases the effectiveness of the support under the longitudinal arch and causes excessive pressure of the tuberosity of the fifth metatarsal bone against the side of the shoe. Pressure concentrated against the fifth metatarsal head causes a sensitive spot to develop over the tuberosity, eventually callus formation at this point, and at times a "tailor bunion."

The inner side of the heel of the shoe may be elevated one-eighth of an inch if inrolling or pronation persists to an undesirable degree with as high a support under the longitudinal arch as can

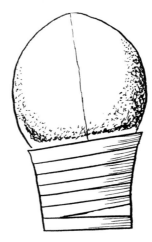

Fig. 114. Position of wedge on the inner side of the heel to overcome inrolling or pronation of the foot.

be comfortably tolerated (Fig. 114). When the inner side of the heel is elevated, a metatarsal wedge should always be used to prevent sliding outward of the foot in the shoe.

An extended or Thomas heel is one which is extended forward one-fourth to one-half an inch on its inner side (Fig. 115). This forward extension of the heel buttresses the shank of the shoes and also gives an upward thrust against the anterior end of the os calcis; this thrust tends to prevent inward rolling of the os calcis and subastragalar joint. An extended heel is very useful in the extremely relaxed type of flatfoot where the thrust of the superimposed weight comes directly on the shank of the shoe, which soon breaks down under the strain and nullifies the effectiveness of the support. The extended heel buttresses the shank and enables it to sustain the additional burden put upon it.

Exercises. If the unbalanced position of the foot has been effectively overcome, the ordinary activities of the patient will usually provide the needed amount of foot exercise. Special exercises to improve the tone of the intrinsic muscles of the foot

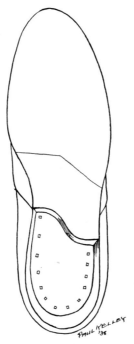

FIG. 115. An extended or Thomas heel which gives added support to the shank of the shoe.

are often, however, helpful. Picking up marbles or jacks with the toes is a very effective way of exercising the intrinsic foot muscles. If shortened calf muscles are present, heel-cord stretching exercises should be carried out; the following is the most useful exercise for this purpose. The patient stands facing the wall an arm's length away. The hands are placed against the wall about the level of the shoulders; the bare feet are toed in slightly and supinated enough to throw the body weight strongly on the outer border. With the back and knees held rigid and bending at the ankle, the patient inclines toward the wall as far as possible by bending the elbow without raising the heels from the floor. A definite and even uncomfortable pulling sensation in the heel cord and calf of the leg indicates that the exercise is being correctly done. This exercise should be carried out ten times night and morning and gradually increased up to twenty-five times night and morning. Additional exercises are described in the chapter on "Exercises."

Physical Therapy. Hot and cold contrast baths and massage are helpful in improving circulation, in relieving muscle tire, and improving the muscle tone.

General Measures. Focal infection and sources of toxic absorption should be removed when present. If the body weight is excessive, a proper dietary regime should be outlined and insisted upon.

Treatment of Rigid Flatfoot

A rigid pes planus or flatfoot is one which is held fixed in a position of pronation or eversion and cannot manually be brought into a position of balance or correction. It is generally useless and extremely uncomfortable for the patient to attempt to correct a rigid flatfoot by the use of supports. Effectively to treat a rigid flatfoot, it must first be thoroughly mobilized by manipulation. The patient should be anesthetized. Manipulation consists of forceful extension, flexion, adduction, and abduction of the foot, repeated until the foot is flexible and flaccid. After the foot joints have been thoroughly mobilized, a plaster cast should be applied with the foot strongly inverted and at a right angle to the leg; the plaster cast should be molded under the longitudinal arch in such a manner as to give as much elevation to this arch as possible. The cast should remain on for from a week to ten days, when it should be removed daily and massage, contrast baths, and exercises used to restore flexibility to the foot joints, the cast being replaced after each manipulation. When the foot can be brought into a balanced position without the use of force, properly balanced shoes with supports should be used to hold it in the corrected position. At times the peroneal tendon and the tendo achillis are so contracted that it is necessary to lengthen these structures by operation before complete correction of the valgus position of the foot is possible. A careful search for possible foci of infection should be carried out and all suspicious foci removed, since infection unquestionably plays a very definite part in the causation of rigid pes planus.

Operative Treatment. While surgery should be used with extreme conservatism in the treatment of flatfoot in the adult, it is the only form of treatment which will relieve a painful foot of the relaxed type which does not respond to careful conservative management. Given a foot of this type, operative correction is justified, particularly in young adults in the active period of life. The surgical procedures most generally used for the correction of adult flatfoot are those of Michael Hoke and Oscar L. Miller which have already been described in detail, page 130. Both these procedures are sound and, when used in properly selected cases and carefully performed, give excellent results. Surgery should seldom be resorted to for the correction of rigid flatfoot and when used it should aim at eliminating painful motion in the subastragalar joint by producing an arthrodesis; attempts to remodel a rigid flatfoot surgically almost invariably fail.

PES CAVUS

(HIGH-ARCHED FOOT)

In pes cavus the arch is abnormally high, there is usually little or no pronation, and the ball of the foot is unduly prominent (Fig. 116).

ETIOLOGY

The cause of pes cavus, so far as the authors' observations go, are, in the main, two:

1. A congenital tendency to a high-arched foot.
2. Unbalanced muscle action.

There can be no doubt but that many persons are born with a foot in which the architectural arrangement of the bones is

such that the foot tends to develop an abnormally high longitudinal arch. When such a tendency exists, the outstanding
feature is usually a plantar fascia which is definitely short and
contracted; often this shortening is so extreme that the plantar
fascia is felt as a thick cord, running across the arch of the foot
like "the string of a bow." Just what the morphology of such a

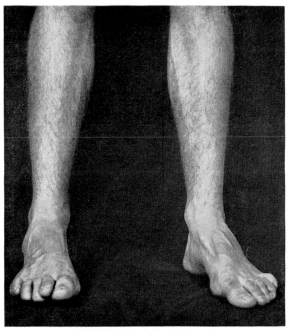

FIG. 116. Pes cavus or high-arched foot. The longitudinal arch is elevated and the
foot tends to roll outward.

congenitally high-arched foot may be is not at the present clear;
possibly it is due to causes similar to those which cause club foot.

The most common forms of unbalanced muscle action which
cause high-arched or cavus foot are a short heel tendon and contracture or overaction of the plantar intrinsic muscles of the
foot. A short heel cord, by raising the os calcis, throws the major
part of the burden of weight bearing on the ball of the foot. This,
in turn, apparently excites a response in the intrinsic muscles of
the foot, and perhaps the long muscles of the leg as well, to meet

the abnormal weight demand. Such increased muscle activity brings about a tightening up of all of the joints of the foot, shortening of the ligaments, crowding together of the bones of the foot, elevation of the longitudinal arch, and prominence of the ball. In other words, the foot under such conditions seems to behave as it does when walking on tip-toe. In fact, the position of the cavus foot is in many respects similar to that which the foot assumes in tip-toe walking. Why a short heel cord should in one foot cause pes planus and in another pes cavus can be explained only upon the basis of fundamental differences in architecture and perhaps a different muscle response. Contracture of overaction of the plantar intrinsic muscles of the foot seems to occur idiopathically in some cases and cause pes cavus gradually to develop; here again perhaps an abnormal architecture may be the underlying cause. Pes cavus also occurs as the result of muscle imbalance owing to infantile paralysis when it is almost invariably due to weakness of the dorsal flexors of the toes and overaction of plantar flexors, plantar intrinsic muscles, and heel tendon. Pes cavus also occurs in spastic paralysis due, however, in this condition to overaction of muscles and not to paralysis.

PATHOLOGY

With pes cavus, the chief disturbance in balance is in the anterior-posterior plane, although a tendency to inversion of the forefoot is seen frequently. At times pes cavus is associated with inrolling of the foot, but such inrolling occurs at the ankle joint, not at the subastragalar joint and is not a true pronation. In the high-arched foot, we have the bones composing both the longitudinal and transverse arches drawn closely together by muscle action and shortening of the ligaments; as a result there is less movement possible in the joints between the bones which make up the foot, and the foot will have less flexibility than the normal or even a flatfoot. The drawing together of the bones of the foot results also in elevation of the longitudinal arch, which is abnormally high. With the increase in the height of the longitudinal arch, the forepart of the foot drops downward, the foot assumes an equinocavus position to a greater or lesser degree, and the ball of the foot becomes prominent. Actual shortness of the heel cord accentuates the equinus; but even if there is no actual shortening of the heel cord, a relative shortening is present because of the equinus position (Fig. 117). It is true that in the paralytic foot we have a cavus deformity developing even with paralysis and

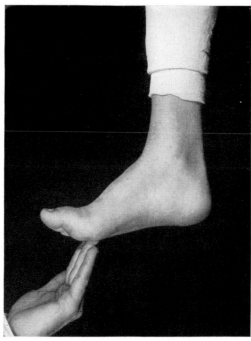

Fig. 117. Showing contracted plantar fascia and relative shortening of heel tendon, due to equinus position of the forefoot.

lengthening of the calf muscles, but this is due to an entirely different set of causes than is under discussion here. Contracture and shortening of the plantar fascia can be demonstrated in practically every high-arched foot to a greater or lesser extent (Fig. 117); in some this shortening seems to be the cause of the cavus rather than the result. In either case, the shortening of the plantar fascia is a very definite feature of the pathology of the high-arched foot. The line of transmitted weight usually falls toward the lateral side of the foot with improper distribution of weight stresses on the metatarsal bones and the entire foot.

The symptoms of pes cavus are those which might be expected from the pathology present, and are both subjective and objective.

Subjective

The chief complaint is usually pain in the ball of the foot, often described as a sensation as if the individual were walking on the heads of the metatarsal bones. There is tiring in the longitudinal arch of the foot, particularly across the dorsum, and cramping in the calves of the legs due to muscle strain and tire is not uncommon. Backache is often complained of. Such backache is due to tiring of the lumbar muscles and ligament strain, the result of the hollow back which is found so frequently in individuals with a high-arched foot. Hollow back is due to or aggravated by a tilting downward and forward of the pelvis, which is brought about by the interference with anterior-posterior balance in these cases.

Objective

The examining positions are the same as those described for pes planus, that is, with the feet parallel and about three inches apart. In the standing position, inspection will show the following: The longitudinal arch is abnormally high, the forepart of the foot is usually somewhat adducted and "toes in" (Fig. 118). Rarely is there pronation associated with high-arched feet; although there may be the appearance of pronation owing to inward rolling of the foot at the ankle joint. The line of transmitted weight usually falls toward the lateral side of the foot, which tends to roll outward.

With the patient sitting, examination will usually yield additional evidence of abnormality such as: The heel tendon is always definitely short, either actually or relatively because of dropping of the forepart of the foot downward. The ball of the foot is prominent, usually markedly so. The plantar fascia is contracted; this contracture can generally be relieved by raising the heads of the metatarsal bones (Fig. 119). Tenderness is present over the plantar fascia and over the heads of the metatarsal bones. Callus formation is usually present over the heads of the metatarsal bones. The mobility of the foot is usually decreased; at least, there is much less flexibility in the foot as a whole than in a normal or a flatfoot unless the latter is of the rigid type.

X-ray yields very little information, but a lateral view will usually show the abnormal height of the longitudinal arch and

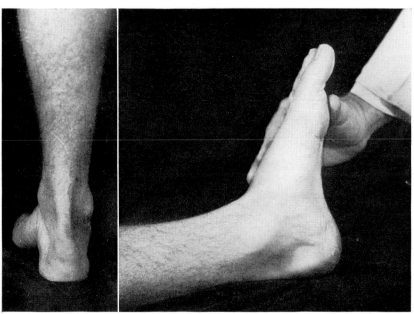

FIG. 118   FIG. 119

FIG. 118. High-arch type of foot. Contracture of the heel tendon, high longitudinal arch and adduction of the foot.

FIG. 119. High-arch type of foot. The ball of the foot is prominent and the plantar fascia is tight and contracted.

depression of the forepart of the foot. An x-ray taken in the weight-bearing position may, however, give important information as to the weight distribution over the foot by showing the comparative development of the metatarsal bones. In x-rays of high-arched feet we have frequently observed definite overdevelopment of the third, fourth, and fifth metatarsal bones, indicating a greater weight strain on the lateral border of the foot than is normal (Fig. 120).

DIAGNOSIS

The diagnosis of pes cavus is based upon the symptoms complained of and on the objective findings on examination. The outstanding complaints are pain or discomfort in the ball of the

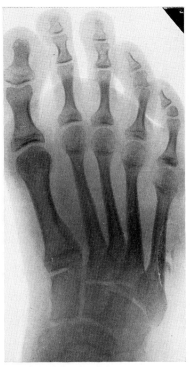

Fig. 120. Dorsiplantar x-ray of foot showing a short metatarsal I and overdevelopment of metatarsals III, IV, and V.

foot and leg tire. Objective findings such as an abnormally high arch, shortening of the plantar fascia, prominence of the ball of the foot with more or less callus formation, the absence of true pronation, and shortening or at least functional shortening of the heel cord, differentiate the cavus foot from the flatfoot and make the diagnosis clear. X-ray of the cavus foot will rarely show structural defects which are so important in pes planus and is, therefore, of minor importance in diagnosis.

The high-arched foot is characterized by an abnormally high longitudinal arch, prominence of the ball of the foot, little if any inrolling or pronation, but rather a tendency to outrolling of the forepart of the foot. With such a foot, the major part of the burden of weight-bearing is borne by the metatarsal arch and the outer side of the foot, as the line of transmitted weight usually falls more toward the lateral side. To bring such a foot into balance and relieve symptoms, we must:

1. Redistribute the weight over the foot so that all the bones of the foot will bear their proportionate part and the metatarsal arch be relieved of the burden of bearing the major part of the body weight.

2. Elevate or restore the metatarsal arch to its normal position; elevation of this arch relaxes the contracted plantar fascia and relieves the heads of the metatarsal bones from excessive pressure.

Redistribution of weight is accomplished by balancing the shoe to alter weight stresses, and the use of a correctly designed support. Elevation of the metatarsal arch is brought about by use of a suitable form of support or by an alteration in the sole of the shoe to be discussed later.

Shoes. A description of a correct shoe is to be found in the chapter on "Foot Apparel," and may be omitted here. One feature of the shoe to be worn by those with pes cavus should be emphasized, however, and that is the height of the heel. The heel cord in the cavus foot is always actually or relatively short, and a shoe with a heel which is too low should not be worn. A low-heeled shoe puts a strain on the shortened heel tendon, increases the burden on the already overloaded forepart of the foot and will usually increase the discomfort already present.

Supports. Supports for the high-arched foot may be of the rigid or nonrigid type. The advantages and disadvantages of each form have already been discussed in the section on Pes Planus in this chapter. The type used is largely a matter of personal preference. While a rigid type of support can be constructed to give support to the metatarsal arch, in treating a high-arched foot, the authors believe that the nonrigid type of support is to be preferred over the rigid type. Accurate fitting and comfortable adjustment of the support used in the treatment of pes cavus is more difficult than is the modeling of a support for pes planus, and it is, therefore, important that the support used lend itself readily to changes in form and height. Experience also indicates that the nonrigid type of support is more comfortable and better tolerated by the less flexible, high-arched foot than is the rigid type. Whichever type of support is used, the particular faults to be overcome must be kept in mind in determining its form and design. The purpose of a support in a high-arched foot is not to overcome pronation and elevate the longitudinal arch as it is in pes planus or flatfoot, but to redistribute weight stresses over the foot and elevate the metatarsal arch; consequently, the support must be somewhat different in design from that used for the correction of pes planus.

RIGID SUPPORTS. Rigid supports made of 19-gauge steel are constructed over a plaster cast of the foot as described on page 164. The foot plate should have the same form as that used for pes planus with some modifications of its forepart. The anterior extremity of the foot plate should be made nearly as wide as the foot and extend forward to the extremity of the sole. As a rule, the forepart of the support should have a greater convexity than is necessary in the plate used for a flatfoot. It is essential that the longitudinal arch be supported as well as the metatarsal arch.

NONRIGID SUPPORTS. Nonrigid supports are fashioned from piano felt and sponge rubber; a number of different types of nonrigid supports have been designed and are in use.

AUTHORS' NONRIGID SUPPORT. The same type of sponge-rubber support may be used in the treatment of pes cavus as is used in the treatment of pes planus (page 173). Such a sponge-rubber support, when used to relieve symptoms in a high-arched foot, should, however, have a different form than that used for flatfoot. Its purposes are the redistribution of weight and elevation of the metatarsal arch, and not correction of pronation and elevation of the longitudinal arch as in flatfoot. Redistribution of weight over the foot is accomplished by making the height of the longitudinal section of the support just high enough to fill in the space between the shank of the shoe and the arch of the foot, so that the entire foot is in contact with the bearing surface and not merely the heel and metatarsal heads. As inrolling or pronation is not a feature of the cavus foot, but on the contrary there is generally a tendency to outward rolling of the foot, an upward thrust against sustentaculum tali is undesirable as such a thrust

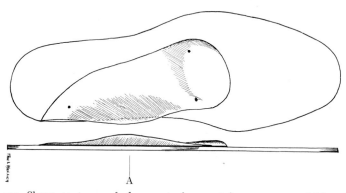

Fig. 121. Shape, contour and placement of support for pes cavus or high-arch type of foot. A, high point of support placed forward.

tends to exaggerate any outrolling present. For the cavus foot, then, the high point of the longitudinal section of the support should lie under the high part of the arch, which is the joint between the scaphoid bone and the head of the astragalus (Fig. 121). The longitudinal section of the support need not extend so far back under the heel for the same reason and so should be shorter than that used for flatfoot. The anterior part of the support is left as high and placed as far forward as the patient will tolerate so that the distal part of the metatarsal bones will be lifted upward, the metatarsal arch elevated, and the metatarsal heads relieved of pressure (Fig. 121).

Both the longitudinal and the anterior parts of the support are necessary to bring the high-arched foot into proper balance and relieve pressure on the heads of the metatarsal bones and the ball of the foot. A short support or pad placed under the metatarsal bones and lacking the section under the longitudinal arch fails in the important feature of distributing the weight over the foot generally, and will, except in mild cases, rarely relieve the dis comfort in the plantar fascia and metatarsal arch. When slippers with extremely high heels are worn with evening dress for short periods of time, a short metatarsal support will often meet the problem of protecting the metatarsal heads and often gives con siderable comfort (Fig. 128).

The method used for accurately placing the support in the shoe and fastening it there has been described in detail in the section on supports in the discussion of Treatment of Pes Planus, page 171, and need not be repeated here.

SHOE ALTERATIONS. In the management of imbalance, the re sult of a high-arched foot, balancing the shoe is often necessary. As a rule, there is a tendency for the foot to roll outward as the line of transmitted weight tends to fall toward the lateral side of the foot. This should be counteracted by placing a metatarsal wedge one-eighth to three-sixteenths of an inch thick between the layers of the sole on the outer side of the shoe with its highest point just beneath the head of the fifth metatarsal bone (Fig. 122).

METATARSAL BAR. Another method of balancing the shoe to relieve pressure on the metatarsal arch consists of placing a bar of leather across the sole of the shoe just posterior to the heads of the metatarsal bones (Fig. 123). With such a bar, the weight when placed on the foot, is transmitted directly to the meta tarsal bones posterior to the heads, and pressure on the heads of the metatarsal bones is relieved. This shoe alteration, sometimes spoken of as a metatarsal bar, is a very efficient device but gives a rather clumsy appearance to the shoe.

Exercises: Exercises in the high-arched foot are useful for two purposes: (1) to improve the tone of the intrinsic muscles which support the metatarsal arch; and (2) to stretch a short heel tendon.

Picking up marbles or jacks with the toes is an excellent exer cise to improve the tone of the intrinsic muscles of the foot,

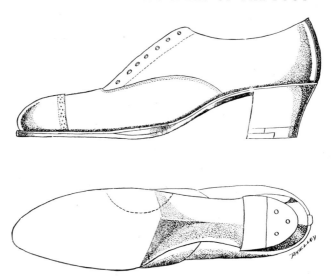

Fig. 122. Metatarsal wedge on the outer side of the shoe sole.

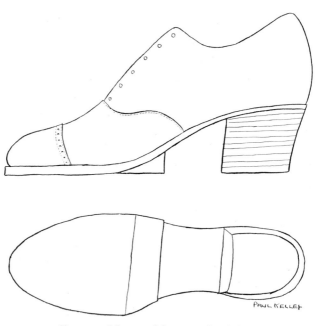

Fig. 123. Metatarsal bar on sole of shoe.

straighten out the toes, and elevate the metatarsal arch. The exercise for stretching the heel cord is described in the chapter on "Exercises"; it may be used to advantage when a contracted heel cord is a part of the pathology.

Physical Therapy. Hot and cold contrast baths and massage may be used to improve circulation, relieve muscle spasm, and build up muscle tone.

Operative Treatment. Pes cavus in the adult should rarely be treated surgically; at times, however, the deformity is so marked and the formation of callus on the ball of the foot so heavy that great discomfort and incapacity result. In this type of foot, if conservative measures fail to give relief, operative procedures should be resorted to. In the adult, stripping of the plantar fascia from its attachment to the os calcis after the manner of Steindler, which is so successful in the adolescent foot, is not as a rule satisfactory since the arch is set in the deformed position and will rarely descend even when the plantar fascia has been relaxed. The most satisfactory operation for the relief of pes cavus in the adult is arthrodesis of the midtarsal joint (see page 143). Sufficient bone should be removed to relax the plantar fascia and allow the forepart of the foot to be brought up into proper relation with the posterior part, thus overcoming the cavus present.

Descent of the Metatarsal Arch and Anterior Metatarsalgia (Morton's Toe)

Depression of the metatarsal arch may occur as a separate entity. As a rule, however, depression of the metatarsal arch is associated with either pes planus or pes cavus; rarely does it occur without evidence of other faults in foot balance. Disturbances of the metatarsal arch uncomplicated are most common in those over thirty years of age, and occur more often in females than in males.

ETIOLOGY

As has been stated, a depressed metatarsal arch is usually due to improper distribution of weight stresses over the foot, the re-

sult of pes planus or cavus. Functional disturbances of the metatarsal arch uncomplicated are as a rule due to a short first metatarsal
bone (Fig. 124), metatarsus varus primus (Fig. 125), or a hypermobile first metatarsal segment (Fig. 126). When these conditions
are present, the head of the first metatarsal bone fails to sustain
its proper share of the superimposed weight which is concentrated

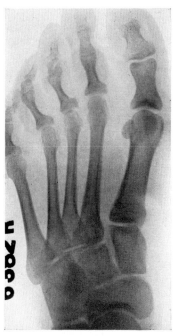

Fig. 124. Dorsiplantar x-ray of foot showing shortness of metatarsal I and overdevelopment of metatarsal II.

on the second metatarsal bone and the three outer metatarsal
bones. Such an abnormal weight distribution brings about an
alteration in the mechanics of the forepart of the foot which, as
a result, is potentially weak. Under the stress of excess use or use
under adverse conditions, such an abnormal or subnormal metatarsal arch gives way and symptoms develop. Unquestionably,
improper footwear plays an important role in the causation of
disturbances of the metatarsal arch. High-heeled, pointed, narrow-
toed shoes throw most of the burden of weight-bearing upon the

metatarsal arch, and at the same time crowd the forepart of the foot and toes and interfere with normal movement and muscle action (Fig. 130). It is this type of shoe which is most likely to

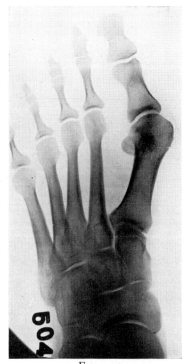 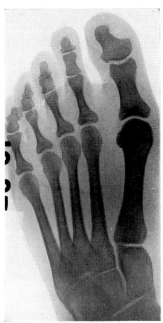

FIG. 125   FIG. 126

FIG. 125. Dorsiplantar x-ray of foot showing metatarsus varus primus.
FIG. 126. Dorsiplantar x-ray of foot showing hypermobile first metatarsal segment

cause a potentially weak metatarsal arch to give way and become symptom producing.

SYMPTOMS

The symptoms of a fallen metatarsal or transverse arch are both subjective and objective.

Subjective. The patient will usually complain of discomfort in the ball of the foot and may state that he feels as though he were walking directly on the heads of the metatarsal bones. In exaggerated cases an acute, cramp-like, burning pain is complained of in one or two toes, usually the second and fourth toes.

Objective. These are usually best examined for with the patient in a sitting position, and are as follows: Loss of the normal dorsal convexity of the heads of the metatarsal bones forming the metatarsal arch; this convexity is usually present, at least, in rest when there is descent of the metatarsal arch. There is nearly always a plantar convexity of the arch so that the ball of the foot is prominent (Fig. 127A). With dropping down of the metatarsal heads, there occurs contraction or drawing up of the toes so that they assume a hammertoe position. Callus formation on metatarsals I, II, and V, or entirely across the ball of the foot is usually present. Evidence of some degree of pes planus or pes cavus is nearly always demonstrable.

METATARSALGIA OR MORTON'S TOE

The condition known as anterior metatarsalgia or Morton's toe was first described by Professor D. P. Morton of the University of Pennsylvania in 1875. Anterior metatarsalgia is due to an insufficient metatarsal arch, in other words, falling or descent of the anterior arch of the foot and represents an advanced form of the ordinary, depressed metatarsal arch. Anterior metatarsalgia is characterized by the sudden onset, usually while walking or weight-bearing, of an acute burning pain, most often in the fourth toe but at times in the second toe. This pain is frequently so severe that the shoe must be removed and the toes massaged and manipulated to relieve the discomfort. Attacks of pain tend to become more and more frequent, and the duration of the pain more prolonged as time goes on. Pain usually radiates toward the ends of the affected toes but may be referred into the metatarsal region of the foot.

PATHOLOGY

From the character of the pain and the mode of onset, it is evident that it must be due to definite irritation of a digital nerve, since no other form of irritation could behave in this particular manner. The explanation of the mechanism of production of

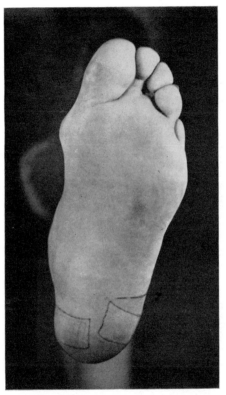

Fig. 127A. Depression of the metatarsal arch with plantar convexity of the ball of the foot.

this pain, which has been accepted in the past, is that with the descent of the heads of the metatarsal bones, the digital nerves come to lie in such a position that if the heads of the bones are crowded together, one or more of these nerves is pressed upon with production of the acute burning pain along its distribution. A similar situation may be produced in the hand. If the normal dorsal convexity of the metacarpal bones is maintained, a considerable lateral compression of the hand can be tolerated without discomfort. If the heads of the metacarpals are made convex toward the palmar surface, a very slight pressure will cause acute pain running into the fingers, owing to the pressure exerted by the heads of the metacarpal bones on the digital nerves. The nerve pressed upon in metatarsalgia is, as a rule, the fourth plantar nerve, which is the most lateral division of the median plantar nerve; this nerve supplies the medial surface of the fourth toe and the lateral surface of the third toe. The fourth plantar nerve is firmly held down against excursions of the toe by the short flexor of the fourth toe, which anatomic fact may produce conditions favorable to pressure on or trauma to this nerve.

Dudley Morton in commenting on the cause of anterior metatarsalgia ascribes the pain to nerve irritation but believes that the irritation is of the median plantar nerve due to an arthritis in the second tarso-metatarsal joint. The arthritis in this joint, according to Morton, is to be attributed to shortness of the first metatarsal with excess strain on the second metatarsal which eventually causes a traumatic arthritis in this joint. While a number of cases of anterior metatarsalgia have been examined in which a short metatarsal was present and could probably be looked upon as the predisposing cause of the nerve irritation, more frequently no shortness of the first metatarsal has been found. It seems then highly probable that while the pain in some cases of metatarsalgia may be caused by irritation of the median plantar nerve, secondary to a short first metatarsal, in others, perhaps the majority, pressure on a digital nerve is the cause of the pain complained of.

Robert T. McElvenny, in an article to be published (Surgery, Gynecology and Obstetrics) and L. O. Betts ascribe the pain in Morton's toe to a tumor, either a neurofibroma or an angioneurofibroma, involving the fourth plantar nerve. When present, this tumor mass lies between the third and fourth toes at the level of the bases of the proximal phalanges, not between the metatarsal heads, and toward the plantar aspect of the foot. Such tumors may result from trauma or irritation of the nerve at this point, but McElvenny believes that the fact that neurofibroma of this nature arise spontaneously at many places in the body must be kept in mind. It is possible that similar tumors may arise at times between the other metatarsal bones, but due to the local anatomy and local application of pressure, these tumors may only infrequently give rise to pain of a severe nature.

McElvenny found a tumor of the fourth plantar nerve twelve times in a series of eleven patients, and Betts in twenty-five to thirty patients. When such a tumor is present in Morton's toe, these observers found the condition to be characterized by intractable pain which does not respond to conservative treatment, diminished sensation on the adjacent surfaces of the third and fourth toes, and at times a palpable tumor between the third and fourth toes where the web joins the sole of the foot. If the toes are dorsally extended, the index finger placed in this location, and a circular motion with firm pressure carried out, at times a mass can be felt, which crepitates and initiates severe pain in the foot similar to the pain of which the patient complains.

TREATMENT

Since the cause of a symptom-producing descent of the metatarsal arch and the more serious condition, metatarsalgia, is improper weight distribution irrespective of the causal factor, treatment to secure relief must bring about a redistribution of the weight so that each portion of the foot bears its proportionate part. Proper distribution of weight over the foot can, as we have already seen, be accomplished only by bringing the foot into a position of balance and restoring or supporting in an approximately normal position the foot arches. Such balancing of the foot can be secured only by correct shoes and properly designed supports with the addition of such other measures as will restore muscle and ligament tone.

Shoes. A correct shoe is described in the chapter on "Foot Apparel," and may be omitted here. It should be stated, however, that if a shoe is worn that is short and narrow at the ball and toe and which has an extremely high heel, relief from metatarsalgia is almost impossible. If a satisfactory outcome is to be anticipated, a shoe must be worn which has adequate room over the ball of the foot and a heel of reasonable height.

Supports. Manufacturers of corrective shoes and many orthopedic surgeons place a small pad of felt or rubber in the forepart of the shoe just behind the head of the metatarsal bones for the purpose of elevating the metatarsal arch and relieving symptoms. While this form of support may work satisfactorily in very mild cases, it is decidedly inadequate in the more severe cases of descent of the metatarsal arch and in true anterior metatarsalgia. A support, to be really effective, must redistribute the weight over the entire foot and support both the longitudinal arch and elevate the depressed metatarsal arch. To accomplish these two purposes a support for fallen metatarsal arch should be of the same design as that used in the treatment of pes planus and pes cavus. The proper shape and height of the support used is determined by the kind of foot present, that is, whether it is a pes planus or a pes cavus, or a neutral foot with little distortion of the longitudinal arch.

Supports may be of the rigid type, made of metal fashioned over a mold of the foot, or a nonrigid type, made of hard felt or sponge rubber. The rigid type of support for fallen metatarsal arch should rarely ever be used unless there is a definite flatfoot associated with it; such a support is necessarily bulky and cumbersome for the amount of correction which is usually required. The sponge-rubber support used by the authors works quite satisfactorily both in descent of the metatarsal arch and anterior metatarsalgia. If a pes planus is associated with descent of the anterior arch, the support under the longitudinal arch should be shaped as described in the section on "Treatment of Pes Planus," page 173, if a high-arched foot is present, the support for the longitudinal arch should be shaped as described in the section on "Supports for the High-Arched Foot," page 190. It should be re-

membered that the anterior section of the support should always
be as high and placed as far forward as the patient will tolerate
comfortably. When a short first metatarsal, metatarsus varus
primus or hypermobile first metatarsal segment is present, a platform placed under the head of the first metatarsal bone should be
added to the support; a platform may even be used alone without additional support in some cases. A platform is made of felt
or sponge rubber three-sixteenths of an inch thick, about one to
one and one-half inches long, three-fourths of an inch broad,

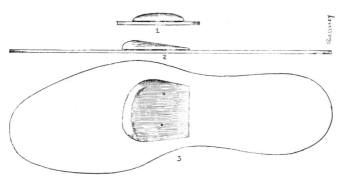

FIG. 128. Shape, contour and placement of support for the transverse arch (anterior heel). 1, anterior view; 2, lateral view; 3, position in the shoe.

placed under the head of the first metatarsal bone (Fig. 128).
Such a platform, by bringing the head of the first metatarsal into
contact with the bearing surface, compels it to bear its proper
proportion of the weight and tends to bring about a more nearly
normal weight distribution over the metatarsal arch. In dress shoes
with high heels it is advisable at times to use only the anterior
portion of the support (anterior heel). (Fig. 128.)

METATARSAL BAR. A very effective method of relieving symptoms due to descent of the metatarsal arch and Morton's toe is
to place a bar of leather one-half to three-fourths inch wide across
the sole of the shoe at the ball just posterior to the metatarsal
head (Fig. 123). Such a bar throws the weight on the metatarsal
bones posterior to the heads and relieves them of pressure. The
chief objection to such a bar is the clumsy appearance it gives the
shoe, and if the same effect can be secured by supports placed

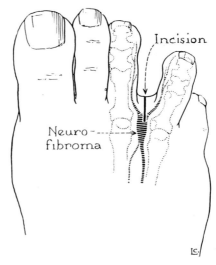

FIG. 127B. Operative treatment of metatarsalgia (McElvenny's operation). Schematic drawing of incision made and location of tumor mass.

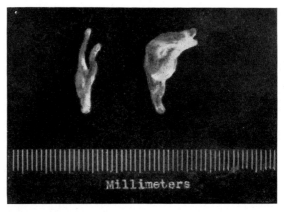

FIG. 127C. Neurofibroma on the fourth plantar nerve removed by McElvenny.

within the shoe, it is usually preferable to use the latter. In severe cases of metatarsalgia, a combination of inside supports and the metatarsal bar have given very satisfactory results.

Exercises. Exercises designed to build up the intrinsic muscles of the foot and overcome contraction of the toes are very helpful and should be used. Picking up marbles or jacks with the toes is a very useful exercise for this purpose. Heel-tendon stretching exercises (page 337) should be employed when a short heel cord is present. A short heel tendon throws increased weight on the already overburdened ball of the foot and interferes with the success of treatment as it makes it difficult to relieve the forepart of the foot of strain by any form of support.

Physical Therapy. Massage and contrast baths are helpful in increasing circulation, relieving spasm, and building up tone in the muscles and ligaments.

Operative Treatment. When acute metatarsalgia is resistant to all forms of conservative management, it may be necessary to resect the head and neck of the metatarsal bone at the point of irritation. The incision for such an operation is made on the dorsum of the foot over the involved toe. The incision passes down to the bone and the necessary amount of bone is resected, leaving the toe in place. It is usually necessary to wear some form of support following resection of the metatarsal head.

McElvenny's Operation. For removal of a tumor on the fourth plantar nerve, Robert T. McElvenny recommends the following procedure: In the first few cases a general anesthesia and a bloodless field should be employed; this makes it easier to locate the tumor mass which is deeply embedded in fat. An incision which splits the web between the third and fourth toes is made. The tumor will be found opposite the base of the proximal phalanges of the third and fourth toes, not between the metatarsal heads, and well toward the plantar surface of the foot. Usually these tumors are fatty and soft on the outside, and firm, white, and fibrous as the center is approached. In the center the plantar nerve is embedded. The largest tumor removed by McElvenny measured 2 cm. long; 1.3 cm. wide, and about 0.5 cm. thick.

Walking is permitted in a split shoe within four to six days after the operation. The stitches are removed on the tenth day. Swelling of the foot is to be expected. Recovery should be complete in five weeks.

Experience indicates that most functional disorders of the metatarsal arch can be relieved by conservative measures. The possibility of a tumor on the fourth plantar nerve should always be borne in mind, however, if symptoms persist after well-planned conservative treatment has been given a thorough trial, and careful investigation carried out for confirmatory evidence if such a tumor is present. If the findings suggest a tumor, exploration and removal are indicated. Resection of the head and neck of the fourth metatarsal bone is seldom necessary or justified.

SUMMARY

In the adult, the foot has taken on its permanent form and to a large extent, at least, has lost its ability to alter its architecture. In the adult, then, little can be accomplished in the way of correcting faults in form and structure, and treatment must be aimed at relieving symptoms. Relief of symptoms is brought about by correcting, so far as possible, the faults in balance present which cause ligamental strain and muscle tire, and give rise to discomfort and disability. A careful examination and intelligent evaluation of the faults present should always make it possible to determine what measures should be taken to relieve a painful foot. Once a plan of management has been determined upon, it must be carried out rigidly if a satisfactory outcome is to be anticipated. Practically every painful and disabling foot disorder can be relieved by proper footwear, proper supports, exercises, and such general measures as are required to overcome systemic factors. The surgical remodeling of an unbalanced foot in the adult should be undertaken with caution and is rarely justified except in young adults in the active period of life, in whom the symptoms are so severe and incapacitating that pain must be relieved and physical activity restored even if surgical intervention is necessary.

10

FOOT APPAREL

Civilization has brought about a very distinct change in the environment of the foot from that in which its development took place. The demands of civilization have removed the foot from an environment of unhampered freedom on the uneven surface of natural ground to one in which it functions on hard, level pavements and floors encased in coverings which materially hamper its freedom of action. That such environmental factors have an important bearing on the prevalence of functional foot disorders is quite evident, since symptomatic foot disorders are rarely seen in primitive, barefoot races. The hard, flat, nonresilient character of the weight-bearing surface upon which the city dweller spends his hours of activity, certainly increases the weight stresses upon the foot and subjects it to greater trauma than does the irregular and resilient natural ground. The coverings which modern life has decreed the foot shall wear interfere with freedom of movement and weaken the structure of the foot to a certain extent by depriving it of the beneficial effect which comes from exercise and free use. The character of the bearing surface cannot be altered, but the character of footwear worn is susceptible of modification along sensible and rational lines. Foot coverings in themselves are not necessarily harmful; in fact, under modern conditions they are necessary; it is the design and fitting of footwear which is open to criticism, and some discussion of this important environmental factor is worthwhile. By footwear, or foot apparel, is meant the hose which cover the foot and the shoes which encase it.

HOSE

The best material for hose is pure silk or wool. Both of these materials are poor conductors of heat and readily absorb moisture. Cotton and lisle on the other hand have a high heat conductivity and do not absorb moisture readily. The weave should be loose and the dyes fast and free from harmful chemicals. Size and elasticity are important. The hose should be slightly longer than the foot and wider than the width of the ball of the foot in weight-bearing. If hose are too short or not sufficiently elastic, they will prevent full extension of the toes, hold them in a cramped position and interfere with their freedom of action.

SHOES

While not admitted by all authorities, it is generally conceded that ill-fitting and incorrectly designed shoes are important factors

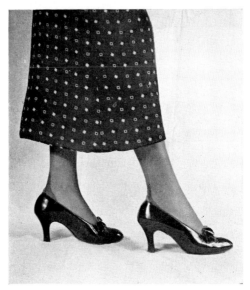

Fig. 129. The type of high-heel, pointed-toe slipper worn by most women—the cause of many cases of foot imbalance.

in the development of functional foot ailments. The feminine part of our population seems to have made style its god and is inclined to follow its every change and dictate. This style worship may be held accountable, in part at least, for a considerable portion of the foot disorders found in women today (Figs. 129-130-131). Children for the most part take little interest in fashion and design; therefore, most of them reach the age of adolescence with feet which have not been abused by wearing improper shoes. During adolescence, girls usually become style-conscious and demand in shoes the latest modes; these, obliging manufacturers willingly provide. The result too often is that before the foot has completely developed, it is subjected to the harmful influence of

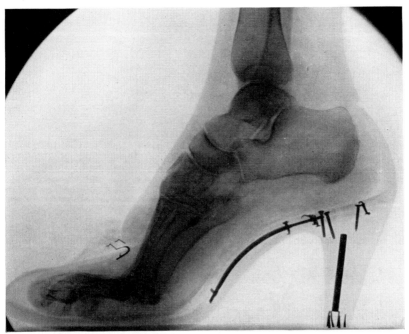

FIG. 130. X-ray of foot with patient standing in a high-heel shoe. Note the position of the foot bones. Patient is compelled to walk on the ball of foot and toes.

shoes which are incorrectly designed or are, at least, ill-adapted to continuous wear. Men and boys are less interested in bizarre types of shoes—in fact, they are inclined to scoff at such oddities; they demand sober, practical shoes built for comfort and wear. It is interesting, in view of these two different attitudes toward footwear, to find that men and boys make up but a small part of the patients seeking relief from foot disabilities—about 8 to 10 per cent.

Much of the criticism directed toward high-heeled, pointed shoes so universally worn by women today should be directed

toward the wearing of such shoes without regard to the work the
foot is called upon to perform while they are being worn. High-
heeled, pointed shoes can be worn intermittently without unfavorable results; it is their continuous use which is harmful. It
is highly desirable, therefore, that for ordinary daily wear a shoe

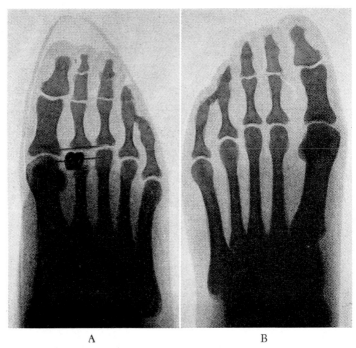

A   B

Fig. 131. Dorsiplantar x-ray of foot. A, with patient standing in pointed-toe,
high-heel shoe (note how the toes and metatarsal bones are compressed); B, same
patient standing in bare feet.

of sensible design which allows the foot to function under a
minimum of strain should be selected. Such a shoe may be des-
ignated as a "working shoe." It is unreasonable to expect our
feminine patients to forego the wearing of style shoes with certain
costumes and on occasions which demand them; all we can hope
for as a rule is a part-time acceptance of suitable or corrective
shoes, and generally this is all that is necessary with a co-operative
patient.

The features of a shoe which are important are the heel, the toe, the sole, the shank, the upper, the lining and the fit. There is, it must be admitted, a lack of complete unanimity of opinion regarding the best type of construction in each of these except

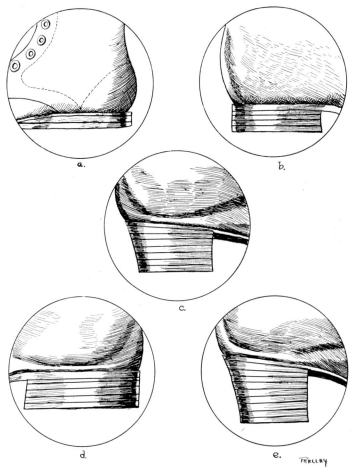

Fig. 132. Correct heel for various types of shoes. a, wedge or spring heel for infants. b, child's shoe. c, shoe for the growing girl. d, boy's and men's shoe e, woman's shoe.

perhaps the toe, the upper and the fit. The opinions on shoe construction expressed here are based on an experience of many years during which shoes of the type to be described have proved the most satisfactory.

The Heel. The heel should be broad enough to give firm support and prevent lateral teetering. The height of the heel varies with the age and sex of the individual. In children, a spring or wedge heel should be worn up to size 8 to 10 (Fig. 132A); beyond these sizes a heel not over three-fourths inch high is correct (Fig. 132B). In growing girls the heel should be broad and one and one-

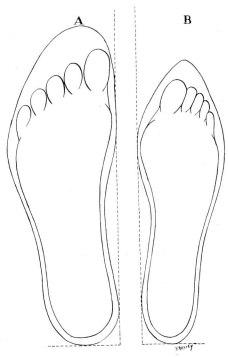

FIG. 133. Sole outline of: A, correct shoe with ample toe room and straight line on the inner side; B, incorrect shoe with pointed toe which constricts the foot.

half inches in height (Fig. 132C) until a shoe size 2 or 3 is required, when the adult height of heel is permissible. Shoes built for women should carry a heel not lower than one and one-half inches and not higher than two inches (Fig. 132E). These measurements will vary with the type and design of the shoe. In men's shoes the ideal height of the heel is seven-eighths to one inch (Fig. 132D). All heels should be of the straight side type.

The Toe. The toe should be shaped to give ample toe room; it should not be extremely pointed but somewhat rounded in shape (Fig. 133). The vamp, that is, the part of the shoe which extends from the upper to the end of the toe, should not be too short; it must be long enough to allow free toe action; the short, so-called French vamp always crowds the toes and interferes with their proper use.

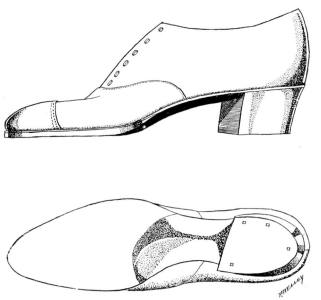

FIG. 134. Proper type of oxford for women. Side view shows cut of upper and height of heel. Lower view shows cut of sole with ample toe room and heel extended slightly forward on the inner side to give added support to the shank.

The cap of the toe should be high enough to insure no pressure on the superior surfaces and ends of the toes. The width of the toe at the ball must be great enough to avoid crowding the foot at this point and allow freedom of movement in the metatarsal region.

The Sole. The sole should be straight on the inner side and on the outer side curve gradually backward, the curve being sufficiently wide to give ample room for the outer toes (Fig. 134) The sole should carry a rather wide shank, yet it should be narrow enough to allow the upper to fit snugly under the longitudinal arch and over the instep. The sole should be narrow enough at the heel to carry a counter which will fit closely around the sides of the heel. The sole should be of the "Flat Sole" type, not the "Rocker Type," and sufficiently heavy to give protection and support to the foot.

The Shank. The shank of the modern shoe should be rigid; and to insure sufficient rigidity, it should be reinforced by a steel shank heavy enough to stand up under the weight of the average individual. This steel shank should be slightly higher on the inner side than on the outer side, should be shaped to conform to the shank of the shoe, and should extend from the heel to the bend of the sole at the ball.

The Upper. The upper should be of the bal- or blucher-oxford, six-eyelet type or high-shoe design. The oxford, if properly constructed, will give ample support for the average foot. Calf, kid or elk leathers are preferable. Patent leather is very hard on the feet because of its lack of porosity.

The Lining. The lining should be of smooth duck, full-lined and free of wrinkles. A careful inspection of the lining of a shoe should always be made before it is worn, as incorrectly cut or fitted linings will produce wrinkles and cause great discomfort, and often render the shoe unwearable.

The Fit. Shoes should always be fitted on the weight-bearing foot. The shoe must be long enough to allow ample room for natural movements of the toes, the tip of the toe-cap extending one-fourth to one-half inch beyond the end of the great toe. The bulge of the great-toe joint should rest over the abrupt curve on the inner side of the sole which is the widest part of the shoe. There must be ample room across the ball of the shoe for normal functioning of the metatarsal arch. The heel should fit snugly and the heel counter should not bulge outward. The upper should lace comfortably and firmly over the instep. If a support or inlay is to be used, this portion of the shoe should be fitted a little larger than ordinarily. The width of the shoe as a whole should be sufficient to permit freedom of movement but not so wide as to allow the foot to shift about inside the shoe.

Common Mistakes Made in Fitting Shoes. The most common mistakes made in fitting shoes are: failure to give sufficient length to allow for the elongation of the foot which normally occurs with use; fitting a shoe too narrow so that the foot is crowded, or too wide so that it fails to support the foot properly; failure to see that

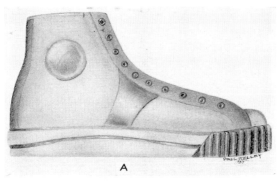

A

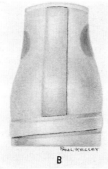

B

Fig. 135. A properly constructed canvas rubber-soled shoe. In A, note the molded sole to support the longitudinal arch. In B, note the tilt of the heel on the inner side to prevent or overcome pronation.

the ball comes at the proper place in the shoe (which in reality means a shoe which is too long or too short); failure to have a vamp of a proper length, i.e., too long or too short for the length of the toes which vary greatly in length even in feet of the same size.

The change from a well-designed leather shoe which properly supports the foot to a canvas, rubber-soled shoe without heel, arch, or adequate supporting qualities such as is used for gymnasium work, tennis, basket ball, etc., is often responsible for acute foot strain which may become chronic. Canvas, rubber-soled shoes designed to give a reasonable amount of support to the longitudinal and metatarsal arches are obtainable in several designs and may be used advantageously by those who wish to take active exercise but are unable to do so because of the foot strain which results when an ordinary canvas, rubber-soled shoe is worn (Fig. 135).

There are on the market today some four hundred and forty-seven different makes of shoes, which claim perfection in scientific shoe building. These shoes vary in makeup and design to an astonishing degree and yet their producers, in most cases, make sensational claims for their efficiency in giving support to the foot and in correcting foot disorders. An investigation of the trademark and trade name registry reveals that nearly two hundred trade names for shoes bear the name of "Doctor." This is, of course, an attempt to capitalize a medical background in the promotion of corrective shoes. The public is very gullible and generally willing to accept the statement that Doctor So-and-So designed or endorses this shoe, without the knowledge or perhaps the will to check the claims made. Unfortunately not all shoes advertised as "corrective shoes" have real claim to the scientific excellency assumed; many of them are the product of a shoe designer's brain or are at the best an attempt to incorporate in the shoe, often incorrectly, ideas, proved or theoretical, which have been suggested to improve its supporting qualities and which in reality have little or no merit. On the other hand, it must be admitted that there are a number of excellently designed shoes for both men and women available today which can be worn with advantage both by those with normal feet and those with symptomatic foot conditions. The difficulty lies in separating shoes with real merit from those which are produced purely for merchandizing purposes and to exploit foot sufferers. The situation is constantly improving, however, for in recent years competent orthopedic surgeons have interested themselves in helping shoe manufacturers who are honest in their desire to produce shoes which are sound in design and have real supporting qualities.

11

HALLUX

HALLUX VALGUS
(BUNION)

Hallux valgus is a deformity of the foot which is characterized by lateral angulation of the great toe at the metatarsophalangeal joint. Enlargement of the medial side of the head of the first metatarsal bone with the formation of a bony prominence which in time becomes covered by a bursal sac (Fig. 136) is usually associated with such displacement of the great toe. The enlargement on the medial aspect of the great toe joint formed by this bony prominence and its bursal sac constitutes what is commonly called "a bunion."

Etiology

For generations, short and pointed-toed shoes have been considered the cause of hallux valgus. While unquestionably improper footwear plays a contributing role in the causation of bunion, its importance has been greatly exaggerated. The basic cause of hallux valgus in the vast majority of cases lies in a weakness or defect in the architecture of the foot. The most important architectural weaknesses which favor the occurrence of hallux valgus are:

1. Metatarsus varus primus.
2. Hypermobile first metatarsal segment.
3. Foot imbalance in the form of depression of the longitudinal and metatarsal arches.

Metatarsus varus primus is an atavistic maldevelopment in which the first metatarsal bone fails to assume the position it should occupy in the plantigrade foot, i.e., close to and nearly parallel to the second metatarsal; it retains, to a large extent, the divergent position which is characteristic of the arboreal or grasping foot. In the arboreal foot, the first metatarsal angulates medially away from the second metatarsal, so that there is a wide angle between these two bones, and a greatly increased interspace (Fig. 137). In the primitive foot, in addition, the first metatarsal bone and its digit are quite mobile and unstable. Metatarsus varus primus, then, since it has all these characteristics, is in reality a throw-back to the arboreal or prehuman foot. Metatarsus varus

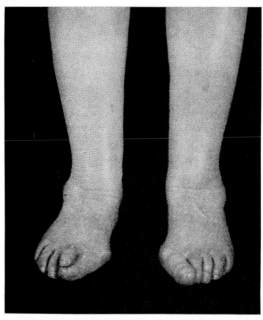

Fig. 136. Typical hallux valgus; showing lateral deviation and rotation of the great toe, enlargement over the medial aspect of the first metatarsal head and hammertoe position of the second toe.

primus, because of the inward angulation of the first metatarsal bone and the associated hypermobility of this bone and its digit, results in a definite instability of the anterior pier of the inner longitudinal arch (head of the first metatarsal) and allows the foot to roll downward and inward, or pronate. The combination of the inward divergence of the first metatarsal bone and the inrolling of the foot produces such faulty alignment of the great toe joint that in walking the thrust of the great toe against the ground tends to force the toe laterally at the metatarsophalangeal joint; in other words, into a hallux valgus position (Fig. 138). Moreover, metatarsus varus primus broadens out the foot across the ball so that it is unusually wide; this broadening of the fore-part of the foot is so characteristic that it has been called a "splay foot" by the British and "Spreitz-fuss" by the Germans (Fig. 139). When such a splay foot is placed in a shoe, particularly if the

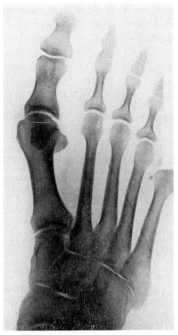

FIG. 137. Dorsiplantar x-ray of foot showing metatarsus varus primus producing a hallux valgus.

shoe is of the pointed, narrow-toed, and high-heeled type, the pressure of the inner side of the shoe against the mobile great toe tends to force it outward; this deviation of the great toe outward is favored by the wide interspace between it and the second toe owing to the divergence of the first metatarsal bone. Numerous observations indicate that metatarsus varus primus is responsible for the development of hallux valgus in the adolescent period in practically every case.

A hypermobile first metatarsal segment because of the increased range of dorsal flexion which it permits in the first metatarsal bone results in the instability of the anterior pier of the inner longitudinal arch; this in turn allows the foot to roll inward, or pronate. The combination of hypermobility of the first metatarsal

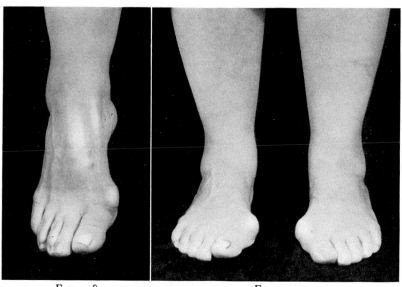

FIG. 138   FIG. 139

FIG. 138. Take-off position showing thrust of great toe against the ground, forcing the toe laterally at the metatarsophalangeal joint, tending to produce hallux valgus.

FIG. 139. "Splay foot," the result of metatarsus varus primus.

segment and inrolling results in the weight thrust falling upon the great toe in such a manner as to force it outward at the metatarsophalangeal joint, i.e., into a hallux valgus position (Fig. 140).

Depression of the longitudinal and metatarsal arches results in faulty mechanics at the great toe joint which eventually bring about stretching and weakening of the structures on the inner side of the joint, and shortening and contracture of the conjoined tendon which is attached to the base of the first phalanx of the great toe on its lateral side. The combination of relaxation of the structures on the medial side of the joint and contracture of those on the lateral side, tends to pull the digit of the great toe laterally and leads to the development of hallux valgus (Fig. 141).

Improper footwear alone may be responsible for hallux valgus in some cases, but as a rule some structural fault with improper distribution of weight stresses on the forefoot will be found if a careful examination is carried out and a dorsiplantar x-ray of the foot is made.

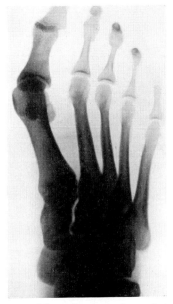

Fig. 140. Dorsiplantar x-ray of foot showing a loose first metatarsal segment and some degree of metatarsus varus primus with development of hallux valgus.

In discussing the etiology of hallux valgus the part played by muscle action should not be ignored. Once deformity has begun to develop, the pull of the extensor proprius hallucis tendon and the conjoined tendon (flexor hallucis brevis and the transverse and oblique heads of the adductor hallucis) tend to increase the deformity through the direction of their pull on the great toe. It is probable, however, that muscle action becomes a causative factor in the production of hallux valgus only after some outward displacement of the great toe has taken place, except when metatarsus varus primus is present.

Arthritis also is responsible for the development of hallux valgus but probably should be looked upon as a contributing factor rather than an exciting cause in most cases.

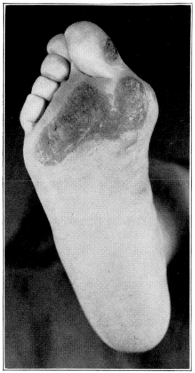

FIG. 141. Plantar view of foot showing depression of the longitudinal and metatarsal arches with development of hallux valgus.

PATHOLOGY

There is lateral deviation of the great toe with shortening of the ligaments and conjoined tendon on the lateral side of the metatarsophalangeal joint of the great toe and stretching of the structures on the medial side of the joint. As the result of irritation of the periosteum by ligamentous pull and friction, an exostosis gradually develops on the medial aspect of the head of the first metatarsal bone. Also due to the irritation, hypertrophic changes and lipping occur about the cartilage margin of the head of the first metatarsal and the base of the first phalanx (traumatic

arthritis). The sesamoid bones become displaced laterally, particularly the lateral sesamoid, and are frequently hypertrophied and
show proliferative changes. The tendon of the extensor proprius
hallucis muscle is displaced laterally, and is usually contracted; in
this position the tendon becomes a factor in the increasing out-

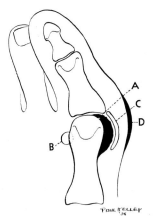

FIG. 142. Schematic drawing of hallux valgus. A, exostosis on the medial side
of the first metatarsal head; B, laterally displaced sesamoid bone; C, bursa over the
exostosis; D, thickened skin over the bursa.

ward deviation of the great toe. In advanced cases, a bursa distended with fluid forms over the prominence on the medial side
of the head of the first metatarsal bone, which from constant irritation may become inflamed and eventually infected (Fig. 142).
A distended or infected bursa may break down and a fistulous
opening discharging bursal fluid or purulent material may then
develop.

SYMPTOMS

The symptoms of bunion are both subjective and objective.

SUBJECTIVE SYMPTOMS

Moderate hallux valgus may cause no symptoms other than the
deformity. The most outstanding subjective symptom is a burning pain at the metatarsophalangeal joint of the great toe. This
pain is caused by pressure and irritation of the prominence on the

medial side of the head of the first metatarsal bone by the inner side of the shoe, or it is due to arthritic changes in the joint. Foot tire and discomfort in the metatarsal arch and metatarsalgia are sometimes complained of, particularly if the hallux valgus is associated with an unbalanced foot.

OBJECTIVE SYMPTOMS

Lateral deviation of the great toe and the prominence on the medial side of the head of the first metatarsal are the most evident objective signs of hallux valgus. Frequently, a hammertoe deformity of the second toe develops due to pressure upon this toe by the laterally displaced first toe (Fig. 136). Depression of the longitudinal arch is frequently present and may be either primary or secondary to the loss of support to the inner longitudinal arch which follows outward displacement of the great toe. The metatarsal arch is nearly always depressed (Fig. 141) and there is pronounced callus formation over the heads of the metatarsal bones, particularly over the second. At times the bursa over the prominence becomes distended with fluid and inflamed and even infected, when it may break down with sinus formation.

TREATMENT

The treatment of hallux valgus should be considered under three heads: (1) prophylactic, (2) conservative, and (3) operative.

PROPHYLACTIC TREATMENT

Faulty architecture of the foot is the basic factor in the causation of hallux valgus in the majority of cases. Probably metatarsus varus primus is the most important structural defect in this respect, although a loose first metatarsal segment and an unbalanced foot due to depression of the longitudinal and metatarsal arches are of definite significance. Such faulty architecture should be looked for in the child's foot and in the foot of adolescence. Much can be done during the growing period to prevent or minimize the effects of these architectural faults by correcting inrolling of the foot, supporting the longitudinal and metatarsal arches, compelling the first metatarsal head to bear its proper proportion of the superimposed weight, by exercises, and by insisting upon the wearing of a correct type of footwear. Correction of inrolling of the foot and support for the longitudinal and metatarsal arches have been discussed in the chapters on "Foot Imbalance in Childhood and Adolescence," as has also the use of a platform to bring the first metatarsal head in correct weight-bearing relation with the other metatarsal heads (see these chapters for the details of the methods used). A straight-last, moderately broad-toed shoe with a heel of reasonable height should be prescribed for feet of this type, and a high-heeled narrow-toed shoe which conduces to the development of hallux valgus should be worn only for dress occasions and only for short periods of time. By carrying out such protective measures as these in the foot of childhood and adolescence, hallux valgus may be entirely prevented or the deformity at least held in check.

CONSERVATIVE TREATMENT

Mild cases of hallux valgus can usually be given relief by wearing a shoe of the proper type. Such shoes have been discussed in the chapter on "Foot Apparel." In addition to wearing the proper type of shoe, correction of depression of the longitudinal and metatarsal arches is helpful in the treatment of hallux valgus, for it relieves the strain on the deformed joint by distributing the body weight more generally over the entire foot. When using supports in the treatment of hallux valgus, care should be taken to shape the support so that pressure on the sensitive bunion will not be increased and cause pain and discomfort (page 167). Manual manipulation to correct the outward deviation of the great toe and the use of pads of felt or of soft rubber between the first and second toes have been used successfully and frequently give satisfactory relief. So-called "Bunion Protectors," made of various materials and designed to be worn over the prominence on the inner side of the great toe joint, often give considerable comfort and combined with a properly fitting shoe and adequate balancing of the foot will often enable the individual with even a marked deformity to carry on quite satisfactorily. None of these conservative measures, however, have much effect in correcting the deformity; and if relief is not secured by their use, they should be abandoned and operative treatment resorted to.

OPERATIVE TREATMENT

The indications for operative interference in hallux valgus are two-fold: (1) A painful hallux valgus which is intractable to carefully carried out conservative measures; (2) an infected bursa with sinus formation.

In planning any operative procedure for the relief of hallux valgus, each case should be considered individually and that operation selected which seems best to meet the conditions present. All operations for the treatment of hallux valgus fall short of the ideal, and all, therefore, require the most careful preliminary study and most meticulous operative technic to assure the patient the best result to which he is entitled. Furthermore, if a hallux valgus is operated upon, it should be remembered that in practically every case, some degree of foot imbalance is associated with the deformity and unless this is carefully evaluated and corrected by balancing the foot subsequent to operation, the result will fall short of what it should be. In other words, the after treatment following operation for hallux valgus is an important part of the management of the condition.

Broadly speaking, there are three types of operation which may be used for the correction of hallux valgus: (1) a type of operation which aims merely to remove the painful and unsightly enlargement on the medial side of the great toe joint; (2) a type of operation which removes the enlargement on the inner side of the great toe joint and in addition corrects the lateral deviation of the great toe; (3) a type of operation which removes the enlargement, corrects the lateral deviation of the great toe, and aims also to correct any metatarsus varus primus which may be present.

Type 1. The first type of operation is satisfactory when there is little outward displacement of the great toe, and the chief discomfort is caused by pressure on the enlargement and its overlying bursa at the metatarsophalangeal joint. Operations of this type have the advantage of simplicity, and if carefully performed in properly selected cases, usually give excellent results.

OPERATION FOR REMOVAL OF EXOSTOSES AND BURSA. A slightly elliptical incision with its base up, approximately two inches long, is made on the medial side of the great toe joint; this incision should be placed well down toward the plantar margin in order that it may be out of the way when healed and not subjected to friction by the side of the shoe (Fig. 143A). The skin flap is dissected well upward completely to expose the bursa overlying the exostosis. A U-shaped incision is then made through the under-

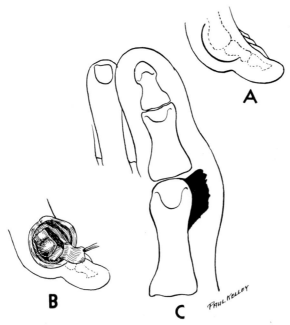

FIG. 143. Operation for removal of exostosis and bursa. A, skin incision; B, subcutaneous flap turned back; C, shaded area indicates the amount of bone removed.

lying subcutaneous tissue, ligaments, and bursa, extending down to the bone and with its base over the base of the proximal phalanx (Fig. 143B). The U-shaped flap thus outlined and including the bursal wall is dissected forward, exposing the underlying exostosis. The exostosis is removed with a thin osteotome and the cut surfaces and sharp edges smoothed off with a rasp (Fig. 143C). If the extensor proprius hallucis tendon is shortened and displaced laterally, it should be lengthened at this point; this may be done through the original incision by undermining the skin. The bursa lining is then dissected from the U-shaped flap and this is sutured back in place under considerable tension to provide a strong internal ligament for the great toe joint. The skin is closed with interrupted sutures, and a dressing applied to hold the great toe in a position of slight inward correction. At the end of two weeks the stitches are removed, a properly fitting and balanced shoe is provided, and activity is rapidly resumed.

Type 2. The second type of operation is necessary when there is serious displacement of the great toe laterally with crowding of the second toe. The Keller or Schantz operation meets the indications for this type of procedure, as it removes the prominence and corrects the outward deviation of the toe without interfering with the weight-bearing function of the head of the first metatarsal bone and is the operation of election. The Mayo operation is extensively used, but in our experience has proved less satisfactory than the Keller type, as it interferes to a greater extent with the weight-bearing function of the head of the first metatarsal. Osteotomy, linear or cuneiform, of the first metatarsal bone has been used to correct valgus deformity of the great toe, but the results have not been generally satisfactory, and this method is not now generally used.

KELLER OR SCHANTZ OPERATION. A slightly elliptical incision with its base up and approximately two and one-half inches long is made over the metatarsophalangeal joint of the great toe; this incision should be placed well down toward the plantar margin (Fig. 144A). The skin flap is dissected up and retracted. A U-shaped incision with its base over the proximal phalanx of the great toe is made through the subcutaneous tissue, the ligaments and the bursal sac down to the bone, and the flap thus outlined is dissected forward, exposing the underlying exostosis (Fig. 144B). This flap should be dissected far enough back to expose at least one-half an inch of the base of the proximal phalanx. The exostosis is removed with a fine osteotome and the cut surfaces and sharp edges smoothed with a rasp. The proximal end of the first phalanx is then carefully freed of all ligamentous attachments by careful sharp dissection for a distance of from one-fourth to one-half inch. The base of the phalanx is then resected with a sharp osteotome and the cut edges properly smoothed; at least one-fourth, at times one-half, inch of the base should be removed (Fig. 144C). The great toe can then be brought into a position of correction or even overcorrection. The U-shaped flap, after the bursal lining has been dissected from its under surface, is sutured back into place under considerable tension and provides a strong

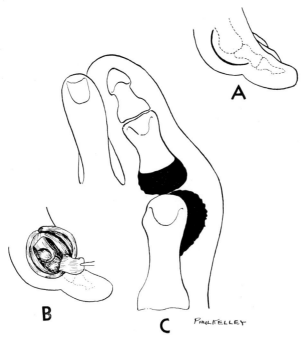

FIG. 144. The Keller, or Schantz, operation for hallux valgus. A, skin incision; B, exposure of joint with subcutaneous flap turned back; C, shaded areas indicate the bone removed.

ligament on the medial side of the joint which holds the toe in its corrected position and insures against any tendency to displacement. The extensor proprius hallucis may require some lengthening in extreme cases; as a rule, this is not necessary. The skin is closed with interrupted sutures. Any form of dressing may be applied which holds the great toe in a position of overcorrection, but care must be exercised to avoid hyperextension of the toe as healing in this position leads to later interference with function and considerable discomfort. The authors prefer to apply mild traction to the great toe immediately after operation, using for this purpose a wire cage over the foot with an extension bar; this traction remains on for about ten days to two weeks (Fig. 145). In a few days, active exercises with the traction in place are started. At the end of two weeks the stitches are removed, a properly fitted and balanced shoe is provided, and use of the foot en-

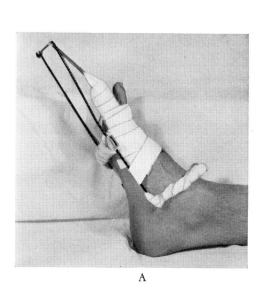
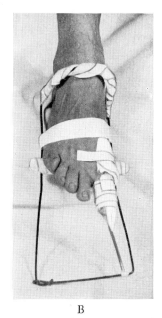

A   B

Fɪɢ. 145. Traction splint applied to great toe. A, lateral view; B, dorsiplantar view.

couraged. Daily, active and passive exercises of the great toe joint should be insisted upon. Normal activity may be started within three weeks and gradually increased.

Tʜᴇ Mᴀʏᴏ Oᴘᴇʀᴀᴛɪᴏɴ. A curved incision is made base down over the inner side of the metatarsophalangeal joint (Fig. 146A). This skin flap is separated from the bursa and retracted downward. A curved incision in the subcutaneous tissue is now made around the bursa with its base forward and left attached to the base of the first phalanx (Fig. 146B); this exposes the joint and the medial exostosis. The distal end of the metatarsal is cleared and dislo-

cated outward, a procedure which exposes its lateral surface. If
the capsule is contracted or tight on the lateral side, it may be
divided. The extensor longus hallucis should be lengthened at this
point to prevent dorsal flexion of the toe. The metatarsal head is
resected by a straight osteotomy, the line being carried proximal to

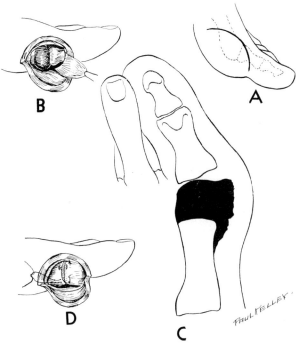

Fig. 146. The Mayo operation for hallux valgus. A, outline of skin incision; B,
subcutaneous flap turned back; C, shaded area the amount of bone removed; D,
the subcutaneous bursal flap turned into the joint and subcutaneous layer closed.

the exostosis (Fig. 146C). The bone edges are smoothed and the
bursal flap which has been dissected back is turned in to the joint
area in front of the bone and held on the lateral side by one or
two sutures. The subcutaneous layer is now turned back over the
joint and the skin is closed. The great toe is dressed in the varus
position and in overcorrection. A gauze dressing or a small piece
of felt placed between the great and second toes and between the
second and third toes will aid in maintaining the position of cor-

rection. The dressing and skin sutures are removed in ten days, and active and passive movements are started. At the end of two weeks, a properly fitted and balanced shoe is provided. Weight-bearing is then allowed. This operation gives excellent results, but the removal of the metatarsal head frequently results in the disturbance of the balance of the foot which may later cause considerable foot discomfort.

Type 3. The third type of operation is indicated when a metatarsus varus primus or loose first metatarsal segment is the primary cause of the hallux valgus. When one or both of these structural defects is present, it is necessary to overcome the inward deviation of the first metatarsal bone in the first instance and its dorsal hypermobility in the second instance if a real correction of the hallux valgus deformity is to be accomplished and a permanent result obtained. The two operations advised in cases of this type are those of Lapidus and McBride.

LAPIDUS OPERATION. The aim of this operation is to produce a bony fusion of the joint between the first metatarsal and cuneiform bones and the adjacent surfaces of the first and second metatarsals and so fix the first metatarsal in correct relationship with the second metatarsal.

A longitudinal incision, five centimeters long, is made on the dorsimedial aspect of the foot; the line of the incision should correspond to the line of the joint between the medial and middle cuneiform bones. The center of the incision should lie over the joint between the medial cuneiform and the base of the first metatarsal. The tendon of the extensor longus hallucis which is exposed should be retracted medially without opening its sheath. The joint between the first metatarsal and the medial cuneiform and the adjacent surfaces of the bases of the first and second metatarsal bones are then exposed subperiosteally.

The tubercle on the base of the first metatarsal bone which impinges against the second metatarsal bone is chiseled off; the plane of the osteotome is held parallel to the long axis of the first metatarsal, and in a strictly dorsiplantar plane (Fig. 147A). The adjacent surface of the second metatarsal bone is roughened with a curette (Fig. 147B). A small wedge of bone is removed from the lateral two-thirds of the articular surface of the medial cuneiform and the base of the first metatarsal; the medial one-third of the joint is simply denuded of its cartilage without removing any bone. The wedge of bone removed should be approximately three or four millimeters at its base, slightly more bone being removed from the cuneiform than from the metatarsal base (Fig. 147B). If too much bone is removed, it may interfere with fusion between the first and second metatarsal bones, and

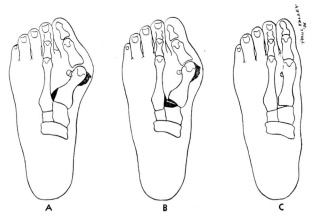

Fig. 147. Lapidus operation for metatarsus varus primus. A, the exostosis of the first metatarsal head and the tubercle of the first metatarsal is removed (shaded areas); B, resection of the first cuneiform-metatarsal joint over its lateral part only. The adjacent part of the second metatarsal base is roughened with a curette. C, metatarsus varus primus and hallux valgus corrected.

between the base of the first metatarsal and the medial cuneiform which is the aim of the operation. After the resection described, the first metatarsal can be abducted laterally without much effort and brought into normal alignment with the second metatarsal, thus correcting the metatarsus varus primus.

A second incision, also five centimeters long, is made over the dorsimedial aspect of the first metatarsophalangeal joint. The medial part of the joint capsule is exposed. A tongue-shaped flap, with its base attached to the proximal phalanx, is made over the medial part of the joint capsule. The bony projection over the medial, and often over the dorsal, part of the first metatarsal head is chiseled off, care being taken to remove all the bony projections interfering with motion of the great toe, especially in its dorsiflexion. The conjoined tendon and the lateral aspect of the joint capsule are tenotomized, if necessary, so that the toe may be brought freely into an overcorrected position, without using force (Fig. 147C). Usually the big toe in hallux valgus has a tendency toward a slight internal rotation, around its long axis, so that the nail is facing medially. A heavy chromic mattress suture is then inserted, first over the plantar distal part of the capsule in front and medially to the tibial sesamoid. The needle is then brought through the dorsal proximal part of the joint capsule and the deep aponeurosis. This suture crosses the medial part of the first metatarsophalangeal joint obliquely from its plantar and distal toward its dorsal and proximal parts.

After tying of this suture, four important points are gained: (1) the big toe is fixed in adduction medially; (2) the internal rotation of the big toe is corrected; (3) the lateral displacement of the sesamoids together with the plantar flexors of the big toe is reduced and this reduction maintained; (4) the deep dorsal aponeurosis with the extensor hallucis longus tendon is pulled medially preventing lateral displacement of the tendon. The tongue-shaped flap of the capsule is then resutured, with the great toe held in adduction, and slight external rotation. The tendon of the abductor hallucis may also be reattached to the medial flap of the joint capsule, thus providing active force, correcting the hallux valgus deformity.

The skin is closed with interrupted sutures and a firm dressing applied, keeping the metatarsal bones closely approximated. In about two or three weeks, a plaster-of-paris cast is applied to the foot, maintaining the correction of the metatarsus varus primus. The great toe is not included in the cast, and active and passive motion is encouraged.

Postoperative care is important. A support under the longitudinal arch should be worn for several months following the operation or until a firm ankylosis between the base of the first metatarsal and the medial cuneiform and between the first and second metatarsal bones has been established. Full weight-bearing should not be allowed before 6 weeks (Fig. 148).

McBRIDE OPERATION. This operation is particularly suitable for mild cases of hallux valgus where the deformity is not extreme and where there are no marked hypertrophic changes in the articular surfaces of the joint.

A slightly curved incision, about two inches long, is made just lateral to the extensor longus hallucis tendon (Fig. 149). The dissection is carried downward along the lateral edge of the joint and the conjoined tendon (flexor hallucis brevis and the transverse and oblique heads of the adductor hallucis) exposed at its insertion on the lateral side of the base of the first phalanx and dissected free from its attachment to the base of the phalanx. The conjoined tendon is then reattached into the dorsum of the head of the first metatarsal bone and held by fine chromic catgut sutures. If the lateral sesamoid is enlarged, it can be resected at this time. The incision is now retracted medially by subcutaneous dissection; the bursa and exostosis on the medial side of the metatarsal head are exposed. The bursa is dissected out; the exostosis is chiseled away, and the bare edges are smoothed with the rasp. The great toe is now manipulated into a corrected position and the capsule repaired. The wound is then closed by layers.

A dressing between the second and third toes will hold the great toe in its corrected position. A light plaster boot is applied. At the end of ten days the plaster and stitches are removed. The toe may now be held in corrected position by adhesive plaster. In two to three weeks a properly designed and balanced shoe is supplied, and activity is resumed.

The McBride operation corrects metatarsus varus by using muscle action to correct medial angulation of the first metatarsal. It is a very excellent procedure for the foot of the adolescent or the flexible type but less effective than the Lapidus operation in the more rigid type of foot in adults.

INFECTED BURSA

In the presence of infection involving the bursa, operation should be postponed until all evidence of infection has disap-

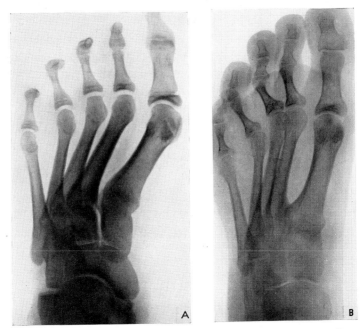

FIG. 148. Dorsiplantar x-ray showing; A, metatarsus varus primus and hallux valgus before operation; B, two years after Lapidus operation.

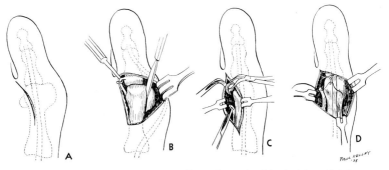

FIG. 149. McBride operation for hallux valgus. A, skin incision slightly curved laterally to tendon of the extensor hallucis longus; B, the conjoined tendon is exposed and severed from its attachment. The exostosis is excised; C, technic of removal of the external sesamoid; D, transplanting the conjoined tendon into the head of the metatarsal. The prominence of the metatarsal head has been removed (From McBride.)

peared. Rest and moist heat are the most effective measures in bringing about subsidence of inflammation and preparing the foot for operation. Plenty of time should be allowed to elapse after complete disappearance of inflammatory symptoms before operation is attempted.

AFTERCARE

Too much emphasis cannot be placed upon the importance of aftercare following operation. Weight-bearing should be permitted and encouraged at the end of two weeks following operation except when the Lapidus procedure is carried out when weight-bearing should not be permitted for four to six weeks. Early and frequent movements of flexion and extension of the great toe joint should be insisted upon. A suitable shoe, properly balanced, should be worn as soon as weight-bearing is started, and its continued use should be insisted upon.

Operations for the correction of hallux valgus have fallen into disrepute among the laity because of unsatisfactory results. Such results are largely due to three causes: (1) failure to select the proper type of operation; (2) failure to carry out the procedure selected correctly; (3) failure to provide adequate supervision of the after treatment and correct faults in foot balance. Selection of the proper type of operation, meticulous attention in carrying out the details of the operation selected and proper postoperative supervision will insure a successful outcome in practically every case operated upon. The operative treatment of hallux valgus is, however, not to be lightly undertaken by those who have not had considerable experience in the treatment of functional foot disorders, for an unfortunate result means, as a rule, a very much dissatisfied patient and much unpleasant criticism.

HALLUX VARUS

Hallux varus is a congenital deformity in which the great toe projects strongly toward the medial side of the foot; it is usually associated with metatarsus varus. The great toe is generally smaller than normal. The extensor hallucis longus and the adductor

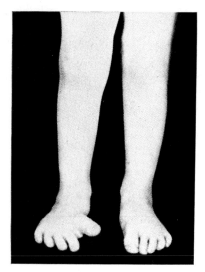

FIG. 149E. Hallux valgus (Haas).

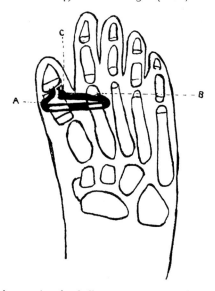

FIG. 149F. Haas' operation for hallux varus. Diagrammatic drawing of the right foot after the second operation, showing the loop of tendons extending around the first phalanx of the big toe and the second metatarsal. (A) Tendon of the extensor hallucis longus. (B) Site of suture. (C) Accessory extensor hallucis longus (hallucis brevis). (From *The Journal of Bone and Joint Surgery.*)

hallucis are usually contracted and hold the toe anchored in the deformed position. The first metatarsal bone is usually short but broader than normal, and the phalanges are usually undeveloped and resemble those found in a supernumerary toe (Fig. 149E).

TREATMENT

In mild cases, a carefully fitted shoe with a platform placed under the first metatarsal head will frequently bring about correction of the displacement as the child grows. With more severe deformity, a plastic operation on the toes or several operations may be necessary, to correct the condition at least to a sufficient extent as to allow wearing a shoe with comfort.

Various operations have been suggested for the correction of hallux varus, none of which has been particularly successful. S. L. Haas has suggested and used the following procedure: An incision is made over the dorsum of the great toe and the medial dorsal aspect of the foot. The extensor longus hallucis tendon is isolated and severed well up in the tarsal region, and the proximal end sutured to the tibialis anticus tendon. The distal end of the tendon is then pulled down to its insertion. All contracted soft structures are divided and the proximal phalanx is lined up with the first metatarsal bone. To accomplish this alignment, it may be necessary to remove some of the head of the first metatarsal and perform an osteotomy of the first phalanx. The free distal end of the extensor longus hallucis tendon is then passed around the medial side of the first phalanx to the under surface of the second metatarsal, and around the lateral border of this bone to the dorsum of the foot. The accessory extensor hallucis tendon (extensor brevis) is then severed at the base of the first metatarsal, and its free distal end pulled over to the second metatarsal where it is united to the free end of the flexor longus hallucis tendon. This gives a strong, tendinous loop, holding the proximal phalanx of the great toe to the second metatarsal bone (Fig. 149F).

The authors have not used this procedure, but since its conception seems sound it should accomplish the correction of the deformity to a satisfactory extent.

TAILOR'S BUNION

Occasionally a bunion develops over the tuberosity of the fifth metatarsal bone (Fig. 150). The cause of such a bunion is pressure or friction over the prominent tuberosity of the fifth metatarsal bone by the outer side of the shoe. A tailor's bunion usually develops in a foot which is broad and splayed out with descent of

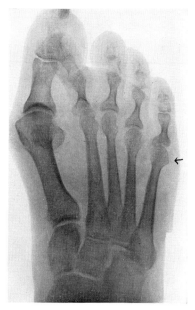

FIG. 150. Dorsiplantar x-ray of foot showing tailor's bunion. Note exostosis on lateral side of fifth metatarsal head.

the metatarsal arch or in a very flat foot with marked pronation. Occasionally there is true outward deviation of the fifth metatarsal bone. These conditions often result in excessive pressure of the tuberosity of the fifth metatarsal against the side of the shoe. The pathology is similar to that of a bunion on the head of the first metatarsal; there is hypertrophy and roughening of the tuberosity of the fifth metatarsal and bursa formation over this prominence.

A tailor's bunion usually responds to conservative treatment in the form of a shoe which is broad enough across the ball to eliminate pressure over the prominence on the fifth metatarsal head and correction of faults in foot balance. Occasionally surgery must be resorted to, and the bunion removed. Removal includes destruction of the bursal sac and resection of the enlarged tuberosity of the fifth metatarsal bone through an appropriately placed incision.

HALLUX RIGIDUS

(HALLUX FLEXUS)

Hallux rigidus is a painful condition, involving the metatarsophalangeal joint of the great toe; it is characterized by a limitation of motion in this joint, chiefly in the direction of dorsal flexion. Hallux rigidus is frequently associated with hallux valgus.

ETIOLOGY

The same factors which cause hallux valgus are responsible for hallux rigidus, i.e., strain on the great toe joint, the result of faulty weight-bearing. Depression of the longitudinal and transverse arches, increased length of the first metatarsal bone, and splay foot all throw the great toe joint out of alignment and subject it to excessive strain in weight-bearing and walking. The resulting irritation excites proliferative changes at the cartilage margins of the joint. Direct trauma undoubtedly plays a role in the causation of this condition in some cases. It may occur as a manifestation of a general polyarthritis.

PATHOLOGY

As stated, the condition is an osteo-arthritis and the joint changes are of a proliferative character. Pronounced osteophytic ridges occur about the head of the metatarsal bone, particularly on the dorsal surface which blocks dorsiflexion of the great toe on the metatarsal head (Fig. 151). Similar hypertrophic changes are found about the base of the first phalanx and sometimes about the sesamoid bones. There is usually a low grade synovitis of the great toe joint.

SYMPTOMS

The most outstanding subjective symptom is pain in the metatarsophalangeal joint of the great toe, aggravated by walking. Since dorsal flexion of the toe is necessary for walking, absence of a useful range of dorsal flexion in the great toe joint throws a strain on the partially ankylosed joint in the take-off position in walking,

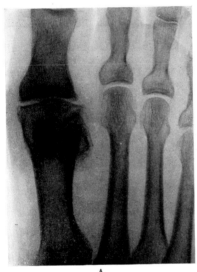

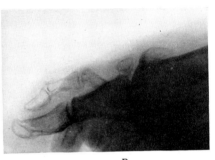

B

A

FIG. 151. A, dorsiplantar and B, lateral x-rays of great toe showing osteophytic ridges about the head of the first metatarsal and the base of the proximal phalanx with narrowing of the joint space.

and pain results. Objectively, there is enlargement of the joint. The movements of dorsal and plantar flexion are limited, particularly the former. In some cases the toe is fixed in plantar flexion and cannot be dorsally extended at all (hallux flexus). Usually an osteophytic ridge is palpable on the dorsum of the great toe joint. X-rays taken in the dorsoplantar and lateral planes will show narrowing of the joint space and hypertrophic changes in the head of the first metatarsal bone and the base of the first phalanx (Fig. 151).

TREATMENT

CONSERVATIVE

In mild cases, relief is afforded by balancing the foot in such a manner as to relieve the involved joint from irritation and strain. This is best accomplished by using a support which holds the longitudinal arch in a correct position and provides anteriorly a support for the metatarsal arch; in other words, the same type of support used for pes planus (page 173). The anterior section of the support should be as high as will be tolerated, for as it elevates the metatarsal arch it raises the head of the first metatarsal bone and allows the limited amount of dorsiflexion present to be used to the best advantage. At times a platform placed under the first metatarsal head accomplishes the same purpose (page 175). A metatarsal bar is also useful in protecting the great toe joint from strain and can often be used with considerable satisfaction (see page 191). A shoe with a rigid sole should be prescribed, as such a sole limits movement in the great toe joint and prevents irritation; such a rigid sole may be reinforced by placing a piece of metal between the layers of the sole under the first metatarsal and its phalanx to act as an additional splint to the joint.

OPERATIVE TREATMENT

Severe and long standing cases with marked proliferative changes about the joint can be relieved only by surgery. Operative measures are of two types: (1) Remodeling of the surfaces of the involved joints; (2) remodeling of the joint surfaces and resection of the base of the first phalanx.

Remodeling Operation. The metatarsophalangeal joint of the great toe is best exposed by the same skin incision as that advised for hallux valgus, i.e., a slightly elliptical incision, with its base upward, placed over the joint but toward the plantar margin. The subcutaneous tissues and capsule are then incised, using a straight or elliptical incision as desired, and dissected away from the metacarpal head and base of the proximal phalanx to fully expose the joint surfaces of both bones. All osteophytes are then removed from the head of the first metatarsal and the base of the first phalanx (Fig. 152), and the head of the first metatarsal re-modeled to provide a satisfactory articular surface. The wound is closed by layers. A splint is applied and worn for ten days to two weeks; the splint should be removed daily after four or five days to permit movements of the joint to be carried out. In two weeks, activity may be resumed with properly designed and balanced shoes.

This type of operation is successful in mild cases in which the proliferative changes have not become too pronounced but should not be used in more advanced cases.

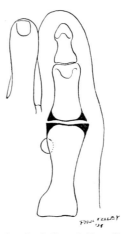

Fig. 152. Remodeling operation for hallux rigidus. Shaded area the amount of bone removed.

Resection of Base of the Phalanx. This is the same operation as the Keller and Schantz operation for hallux valgus (page 226). The skin incision is the same as the one used in the Keller opera-tion. The skin is dissected back, exposing the subcutaneous tissue and internal lateral ligament. A U-shaped flap with its base over the proximal end of the phalanx and including the subcutaneous tis-sues down to the bone is then outlined; this flap should be dis-sected free and far enough distally to expose at least one-fourth to one-half inch of the proximal end of the phalanx. Osteophytes and the hypertrophic ridge are removed from the head of the metatarsal bone and the joint surface is remodeled, leaving a small area of cartilage on the end of the bone. The base of the proximal phalanx is then carefully cleared of all ligamentous and tendinous attachments, and one-fourth to one-half inch of the base is resected (Fig. 153). The amount of bone removed depends upon the severity of the condition; if there is marked limitation of motion with excessive narrowing of the joint space, at least one-half inch of bone must be removed if useful and pain-free motion is to be expected. If the sesamoids, particularly the lateral sesamoid, are enlarged and irregular, one or both of these should be removed.

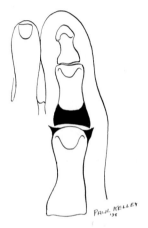

FIG. 153. Resection of base of proximal phalanx for hallux rigidus. Shaded area the amount of bone removed.

After-treatment consists of immobilization for two weeks. The authors prefer traction to provide immobilization for a period of ten days, using a wire cage over the foot with a traction arm and rubber elastic (Fig. 145). Traction keeps the bone ends apart and favors the formation of a satisfactory joint space as the tissues contract down. Daily movement should be instituted after one week. Activity may be resumed in two to three weeks in a properly designed and balanced shoe.

The results of the operative treatment for hallux rigidus should be excellent provided the procedure selected is the one indicated in the particular case operated upon, the operation carefully performed, and the after-treatment carefully supervised.

HAMMERTOE

Hammertoe is a deformity of one or more toes of the foot, characterized by a dorsiflexion of the metatarsophalangeal joint, acute plantar flexion and rigidity of the midphalangeal joint, and extension at the distal phalangeal joint. In certain cases, the distal joint remains straight and the tip of the toes impinge on the ground; this type is sometimes called "mallet toe." Any or all of the toes may be involved but the second toe is most frequently affected (Fig. 154).

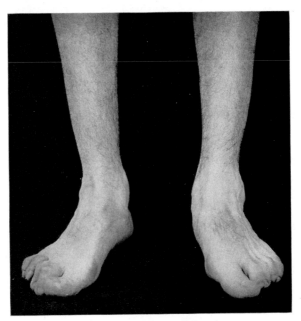

Fig. 154. Hammertoe deformity.

Etiology

Some cases of hammertoe are definitely congenital. Congenital hammertoe usually involves the second or fifth toe; such congenital hammertoes are usually a familial characteristic. Acquired hammertoe is usually secondary to faulty foot balance, particularly descent of the metatarsal arch. Multiple hammertoes, not the result of paralysis, are usually associated with an extremely high-arched or claw foot. Improper footwear is undoubtedly an important contributing cause, particularly high-heeled, sharp-pointed, and short shoes, which hold the toes in a cramped position. Hammertoe involving the second toe is frequently associated with hallux valgus.

PATHOLOGY

The deformity of the toe is essentially a contracture of the plantar fibers of the lateral ligaments and particularly the glenoid ligament at the proximal phalangeal joint. The long tendons of the toe play no material part in causing the deformity but become secondarily shortened. The midphalangeal joint becomes enlarged and a bursa or corn usually develops over the prominence of the joint.

SYMPTOMS

The outstanding subjective symptom is pain and sensitiveness over the prominent toe joint. Objectively, there is deformity of the toe and bursa formation over the prominence; this latter may become inflamed or infected. In "mallet toe," a callosity frequently forms over the end of the toe in close proximity to the nail which becomes very sensitive.

TREATMENT

CONSERVATIVE

Numerous methods of padding and splinting hammertoes have been suggested; but as a rule, they are very unsatisfactory. In mild cases, proper shoeing and elevation of the depressed metatarsal arch by a properly designed support (page 200) will often afford relief and bring about a measure of correction of the toe deformity. Such conservative measures should be thoroughly followed out in mild and early cases. When a marked hammertoe has developed with bursa formation, operative interference is usually necessary for relief.

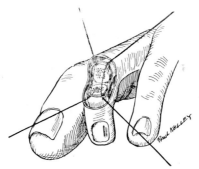

FIG. 155A. Schematic drawing of operation for the correction of hammertoe deformity.

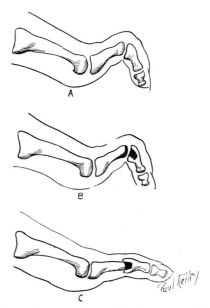

FIG. 155B. (A) Lateral view of bones in hammertoe. (B) Head of proximal phalanx and base of the middle phalanx shaped by operation. (C) Shaped head of middle phalanx fitted into cavity in base of middle phalanx. (Redrawn from *The Journal of Bone and Joint Surgery.*)

OPERATION

The only effective operation for the correction of hammertoe consists in resection of the proximal interphalangeal joint with or without the removal of the overlying bursa.

A transverse elliptical incision over the prominence of the interphalangeal joint may be used. This incision removes a small ridge of skin and at the same time the corn and its underlying bursa. The long extensor tendon is cut across, completely exposing the joint. Division of the tendon is not important since the aim of the operation is to produce ankylosis of the joint and the tendon is of little use. A curved, longitudinal incision with lateral retraction of the tendon may be used, however, as a method of approach. The joint is entered after division of the capsule, and the head of the proximal phalanx and the base of the middle phalanx are cleared of soft tissue back for a distance of approximately one-fourth inch. The head of the proximal phalanx and the base of the middle phalanx are then resected; sufficient bone should be removed to allow the toe to come completely straight (Fig. 155A). One or two catgut sutures passed through the severed ends of the branch of the extensor longus tendon will hold the denuded bone surfaces firmly in place and prevent displacement. A splint should be worn for four to six weeks or until complete ankylosis takes place.

Young Operation for Hammertoe. Charles S. Young has suggested a modification of the Higgs technic for the correction of hammertoe as follows:

Through a short linear incision over the dorsal aspect of the metatarsophalangeal joint, a tenotomy of the long and short extensors of the toe is performed. In severe cases, it is necessary to incise a tight fibrous band, which extends across the dorsum of this joint. In the operation on the toe itself, a linear incision is made over the proximal phalangeal joint, medial or lateral to the extensor tendon, so placed as to avoid the digital artery. The expansion of the long extensor tendon is exposed and divided transversely, one-half centimeter proximal to the joint. The distal end is reflected forward to expose the joint surface. The distal extremity of the proximal phalanx is dissected free of soft parts, sufficiently to expose the head and a fourth of the shaft of the bone. By means of a small, dental rongeur forceps, the cartilage is excised from the head of the proximal phalanx, and the end of the bone is reshaped to resemble a truncated cone. It is important not to remove the distal cortex, since it is necessary to preserve this to maintain the required strength of the bone. This is the one point in which Young differs from the Higgs technic. A drill hole is made in the joint surface of the base of the second phalanx, penetrating to the marrow cavity; this drill hole is gently enlarged with a small gouge until a cavity is secured into which the pointed end of the first phalanx will snugly fit. The pointed end of the first phalanx is fitted firmly into the cavity, care being taken properly to align the phalanges to avoid later deformity (Fig. 155B). The dorsal expansion of the extensor tendon is sutured, and the wound is closed in layers. A splint is worn from three to four weeks.

When the fifth toe is involved, amputation of the toe is the most effective method of treatment. When the fifth toe is amputated, the distal end of the fifth metatarsal bone should be removed. This gives a better shape to the foot, but, more important, it serves to minimize the danger of a hammertoe developing in the fourth toe—a not infrequent occurrence when the fifth toe alone is removed. Resection of the proximal phalangeal joint is unsuccessful, since ankylosis practically never takes place. Amputation of any toe other than the fifth for hammertoe should not be performed; this is particularly true in regard to the second toe. Amputation of the second toe nearly always leads to a wandering outward of the great toe and hallux valgus deformity.

Tenotomy of the long extensor tendon (an operation frequently performed) does not correct hammertoe and in fact may do harm by allowing further dorsiflexion of the proximal phalanx. Division of the long extensor tendon fails to permanently cure a true hammertoe because the structures responsible for the deformity are the interphalangeal ligaments as has been pointed out in the paragraph on "Pathology"; the long extensor tendon is involved only secondarily. Unless the contractures of the interphalangeal ligaments are overcome, deformity will recur.

Contractures of all the toes resulting from the extreme muscle imbalance such as is encountered in poliomyelitis or in spastic paralysis do not fall within the scope of this work.

INJURIES TO THE SESAMOID BONES

The sesamoid bones of the foot, particularly those beneath the metatarsophalangeal joint of the great toe, are often irritated or injured, and occasionally fractured (Fig. 156).

Improper weight-bearing with concentration of weight on the head of the first metatarsal bone may cause a localized irritation of the sesamoid bones of the great toe joint; along with this irritation a condition resembling a bursitis may develop. Long-continued irritation may cause proliferative changes to take place in the sesamoids which increase in size and become irregular in shape; exostoses may even be felt about the margins of such an irritated sesamoid. Irritation of a sesamoid is characterized by local pain over the involved bone and tenderness at the same point.

TREATMENT

The treatment of irritation or bursitis involving a sesamoid bone consists of relief from pressure and the impact of weight-bearing. This is most effectively accomplished by placing a support in the shoe to protect the forepart of the foot from contact with the ground. The type of sponge-rubber support described on page 201 may be readily shaped to accomplish this purpose. Felt and sponge-rubber pads of various shapes may also be used. If the condition is extremely acute, complete rest and local heat will quiet down the acute process. When conservative measures fail to give relief, and the painful condition persists, resection of the sesamoid is indicated. Resection of a sesamoid bone should be done carefully with as little damage as possible to the tendon in which it is embedded.

Fracture of the sesamoid bone of the great toe may occur as the result of trauma, usually a direct impact on the bone. Fracture of one or both sesamoids of the great toe usually results, however, from violent muscular action. Such a fracture occurred on two occasions in professional baseball players while making a sudden, violent effort to start quickly. Fracture of a sesamoid is characterized by the sudden onset of acute pain following injury, localized on the plantar surface of the great toe joint. The pain and disability tend to continue and cause interference with the use of the foot for some time. The diagnosis is made on the history, the local pain and tenderness, and x-ray evidence of

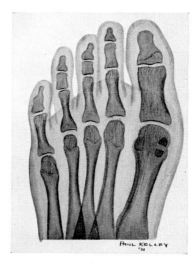

FIG. 156. Tracing of dorsiplantar x-ray showing a fracture of the medial sesamoid of the first metatarsal.

fracture. Sesamoid bones are often bipartite, and this developmental variation must be borne in mind in interpreting the x-ray plates. As a rule, the regular outline and clear cut margins of the bipartite bones will serve to distinguish them from fractures.

A fractured sesamoid bone should be treated by rest and protection from weight-bearing until healing has occurred. A plaster cast from the knee to the toes may be applied and worn for from two to three weeks. Such immobilization should be followed by the use of a support which will protect the forepart of the foot from the trauma of weight-bearing. Convalescence from this injury is usually slow, and healing requires a number of weeks. Excision of a fractured sesamoid is indicated if symptoms and disability persist in spite of conservative treatment.

12

AFFECTIONS OF THE NAILS

INGROWING TOE NAIL

(Onychocryptosis—Onychia)

Onychocryptosis, commonly called ingrowing toe nail, is an affection in which there is an acute inflammatory reaction, often frank infection, of the soft tissues at the corner of the nail of a toe. The nail of the great toe is most often involved.

ETIOLOGY

While there are a number of contributing factors which cause ingrowing toe nail, faulty foot balance which throws a distorting

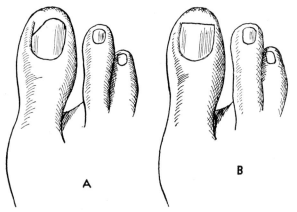

FIG. 157. Trimming of nails. A, improper trimming; B, proper trimming of the toe nail with square corners.

stress on the great toe is by far the most important direct cause. If careful observation of the stance of the foot is made in individuals complaining of ingrowing toe nails, faulty foot balance will usually be found. In addition, short, pointed shoes which make pressure on the nail of the great toe, careless and improper trimming of the nails, and excessive width and abnormal convexity of the nail result in local irritation and eventually cause an ingrowing nail (Fig. 157).

SYMPTOMS

Pain, tenderness, swelling, and redness at the corner and along the lateral margin of the nail characterize the affection. Frequently there is frank infection of the involved area with pus formation, following which the skin breaks down and a discharging area covered with sluggish granulations develops.

TREATMENT

CONSERVATIVE

Mild ingrowing toe nail is best treated by prescribing the proper type of shoe, correcting faulty foot balance, and packing the nail

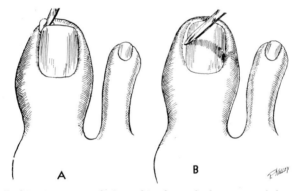

FIG. 158. Packing ingrown nail. A, packing beneath the corner of the nail; B, packing the nail fold away from the nail.

with cotton. When packing a nail, a fine film of cotton should be inserted along the sides of the nail and under the corners. The corner of the nail is usually turned down and forms a sharp spike-like projection which is deeply embedded in inflamed soft tissue. Packing cotton under the corner of the nail lifts up the turned down edges and relieves the underlying soft parts of pressure and irritation (Fig. 158). If packing is continued for several weeks, as the nail elongates, it tends to grow in a more normal direction and away from the irritated soft tissues. The common mistake made in packing a nail is to use too much cotton, which wads up and causes pain and discomfort. If infection and redundant granulations are present, the cotton packing is saturated with a 10 per cent solution of silver nitrate for several packings; this rapidly destroys the excess granulations and clears up the infection.

OPERATIVE TREATMENT

An ingrowing toe nail which fails to respond to conservative measures can be relieved only by operation. Any operation which is to be successful must remove a sizeable section of the nail including its matrix. Removal of the entire nail is an operation which is rarely successful and even more rarely indicated.

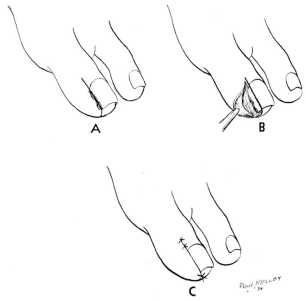

Fig. 159. Operation for excision of ingrowing toe nail. A, line of incision for the skin flap; B, skin flap retracted and line of incision for excision of nail portion and subcutaneous tissue; C, incision closed.

Technic of Operation. An incision is made along one or both sides of the nail to be operated upon, extending from the anterior margin of the nail well back of the matrix. This incision includes the entire thickness of the soft parts and outlines a flap which is turned completely back, exposing the margin of the nail throughout its extent (Fig. 159A). A second incision is made parallel to the first and placed closely alongside the distal phalanx; this second incision removes a generous section of the nail, all the soft parts down to the plantar surface of the toe, and the matrix of the section of the nail which is removed (Fig. 159B). The original flap is then sutured snugly back into place with a few interrupted sutures (Fig. 159C). This operation reduces the width of the nail, removes the rough nail margin, destroys the matrix of the section of the nail removed, and eliminates redundant soft parts. This has proved to be the most satisfactory operation for ingrowing nail in the authors' experience.

CLUB NAIL

(Onychogryposis)

Club nail, or onychogryposis, is a condition of excessive hypertrophy of the nail generally appearing in the nails of the toes, although the same affection but of a lesser degree is often found in the nails of the hands (Fig. 160A). The nail of the great toe is most frequently affected although, in some cases, all the toes of the foot may show this unusual thickening.

The twisted and thickened nail is generally found in the aged and is thought to be due to an irritation or pressure on the nail end, which in turn irritates the matrix which causes the nail to grow unevenly and at an increased rate. The dorsal layers grow more profusely than do the plantar, hence the end of the nail curls downward and the dorsal layers pile up to form a horn-like structure.

The treatment consists in clipping the nail short with heavy bone shears. This will give temporary relief, but the overgrowth of nail generally continues. It is often advisable to soften the nail with salicylic acid or calcium sulphide before clipping.

When the club nail is sufficiently enlarged to be a source of constant trouble by wearing holes in the hose or making the wearing of a shoe uncomfortable, it should be removed. A very satis-

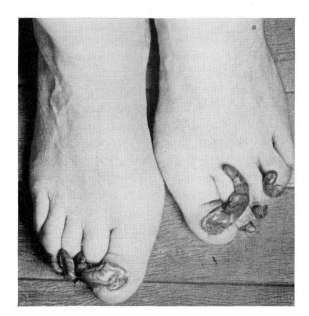

FIG. 160A. Club nails.

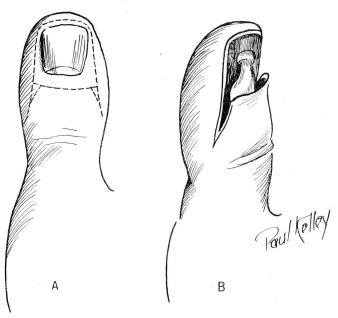

FIG. 160B. (A) Skin incision. (B) Nail and nail bed completely removed.

factory result can be obtained by the removal of the nail, including complete removal of the matrix; unless the entire matrix is removed, the nail will return.

Removal of the nail is best accomplished by a U-shaped incision, surrounding the nail and dissecting out the entire nail with its matrix (Fig. 160B). A careful closure will reduce the area uncovered by skin; the exposed area is allowed to granulate over. In extreme cases, the distal half of the last phalanx may be resected or the toe amputated through the distal joint.

13

AFFECTIONS OF THE SKIN

CALLUS AND CORNS—CLAVUS

A callus is a localized horny thickening of the epidermis which forms over an area of the foot or toes subjected to pressure or

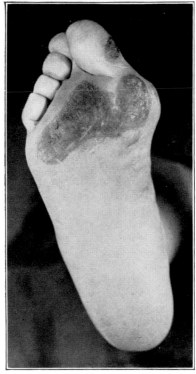

FIG. 161. Callous formation on the ball of the foot resulting from abnormal pressure by the heads of the metatarsal bones.

friction which normally is not exposed to pressure. Such pressure, when it occurs over prominences which afford counter-pressure, sets up a local irritation as the result of which there is a proliferation of the epidermis and callus formation (Fig. 161). In certain areas, particularly the dorsal surface of the midphalangeal joints of the toes, and the lateral surface of the fifth toe, the proliferating horny layer of the skin tends to draw up in concentric layers so that a conical mass is produced which is broad and flat at the surface and tapers to an apex which extends deep into the papillae of the corium; this constitutes a corn or clavus (Fig. 162).

ETIOLOGY

Corns may develop spontaneously, but as a rule they are the result of pressure and friction from ill-fitting shoes, particularly

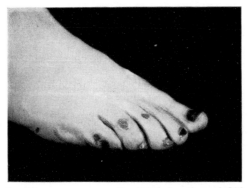

FIG. 162. Clavus or corn on the third, fourth, and fifth toes.

short, narrow-toed shoes, which crowd the toes together and force them into a hammertoe position. Hammertoe itself is a cause of corn formation. Faulty foot posture with concentration of weight stresses on certain areas of the foot is another causative factor. Small exostoses at the joint margins of the interphalangeal joints cause clavus formation from pressure upon an adjoining toe.

SYMPTOMS

As the horny layers of the corn become thickened, the apex is forced deeper into the sensitive papillae of the corium, and discomfort and pain result. Objectively, there is a circumscribed callus, which when trimmed away reveals a horny mass extending as a cone downward into the deeper areas.

TREATMENT

CONSERVATIVE

Proper shoes and the correction of faulty foot balance are the first requisite of treatment; most corns will disappear spontaneously if pressure is removed. When a corn is well developed, local treatment is necessary. The hard, bony plate should be removed with a razor blade or the foot soaked in hot water and the excess epithelium removed by rubbing with fine sandpaper. After the removal of the base of the corn, salicylic acid in flexible collodion should be applied to the surface; this will soften the corn and, after a few applications, it can be picked or soaked off. The following prescription is very effective for this purpose:

℞

Acid Salicylic	1.
Ext. Cannabis Indica	.50
Ether	3.
Flexible Collodion	
Q. S. AD.	10.

Apply with applicator or camel's hair brush.

OPERATIVE TREATMENT

Persistent corns which do not disappear with such conservative measures require surgical removal. There is usually a bursal formation which has developed beneath the corn, and a small exostosis is probably present.

Walter I. Gelland advises the following technic: The toe is anesthetized with 2 per cent procaine hydrochloride. It is most advisable to use a regional anesthetic introduced at the base of the toe, so that the area of the corn should not be infiltrated. After the foot has been properly prepared, the thickened epithelium is removed from the corn by means of a sharp curette. If the operator begins to dissect with the curette around the margins of the corn, he will be able to find a natural plane of cleavage between the thickened and the normal skin, and the entire superficial structure of the corn can be removed en masse. The area of the corn is outlined with a semi-elliptical incision and the skin is dissected back. A bursal structure underlying the flap will now be found overlying the interphalangeal joint and above the extensor tendons. The bursa is dissected out and removed. The extensor tendons are displaced laterally or medially, and the joint margins are inspected. Any bony prominence present can usually be delineated or can be found by digital inspection. The prominence can be removed with a small chisel or long shear. The wound is closed with silk sutures which may be removed at the end of a week. The patient should be kept off his feet for two or three days.

SOFT CORNS

Soft corns occur on the lateral surfaces of and in the web between the toes, from pressure. As such soft corns lie between the toes, they do not become hard and dry but are soft and elastic because of moisture and maceration; for this reason, they are called "soft corns." Such soft corns are caused by pressure of a toe against a neighboring toe and are very difficult to eradicate. While unquestionably crowding of the toes together by ill-fitting shoes does cause a soft corn, many of them are due to pressure of the toe against a bony prominence on the opposing toe. Most soft corns occur between the fourth and fifth toes, and the bony prominence is, according to Albert Key, nearly always on the base of the first phalanx of the fourth toe.

TREATMENT

The majority of soft corns will disappear if a properly designed and fitted shoe is worn and faulty foot balance is corrected. In correcting faulty balance, particular care must be directed toward elevating the metatarsal arch as elevation of this arch separates the toes from each other. This separation of the toes overcomes the crowding of one toe against the neighboring toe. If a soft corn does not disappear with correction of faulty foot balance and proper shoeing, it is probably the result of pressure against a bony prominence, and this prominence must be removed if relief is to be given.

Albert Key recommends the following procedure: An incision is made on the lateral side of the dorsum of the fourth toe near its base. This is carried down to the bone, the dissection being medial to the small artery and nerve on the lateral side of the toe; the incision extends a short distance upward on the dorsum of the foot. With a small retractor, tissues are drawn outward, and the lateral surface of the proximal portion of the shaft and the base of the first phalanx of the fourth toe are exposed. With a small chisel the lateral portion of the base is cut off flush with the shaft, thus removing about one-fourth of the base of the phalanx (Fig. 163). After it is cut off, the fragment of bone is

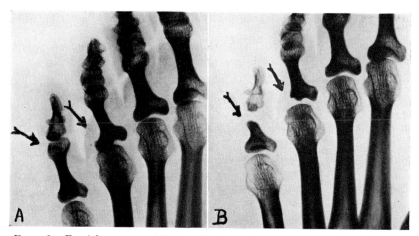

Fig. 163. Dorsiplantar x-ray of toes showing: A, exostosis on phalanges which causes irritation and corns; B, after the removal of the exostosis. (Courtesy, A. Key.)

cut loose from the joint capsule and removed. Care is taken not to injure the cartilage on the head of the fourth metatarsal, and no attempt is made to close the joint or the joint capsule. The deep structures are closed with two or three sutures of ooo catgut, and the skin is closed with silk. The toe is not splinted, but is incompletely immobilized in a small dressing of gauze and adhesive. The patient remains off his feet for two or three days, occasionally a week, and after this normal activity of the foot can be resumed.

VERRUCA PLANTARIS

Plantar warts are small circumscribed callus-like growths which form on the plantar surface of the foot and about the heel. Plantar warts are often confused with callosities and corns, but they differ materially from these conditions. If the top of a plantar wart is removed by shaving off the horny callous layer with a sharp razor blade, a central core composed of hypertrophied papillae, which is soft and vascular and has a marked tendency to bleed, will be found (Fig. 164).

ETIOLOGY

The etiology of plantar warts is not known, although Kuhnemann describes a bacillus which is believed to be etiologic. Certainly, plantar warts are infectious in origin; and, once infection has occurred, they tend to spread to other parts of the foot. The presence of an area of lowered resistance, such as a callosity, is a

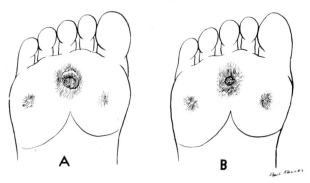

FIG. 164. Verruca plantaris or plantar wart. A, the wart appears as a heavy callus; B, after the top has been trimmed off the central core is evident.

strong predisposing factor—in fact, plantar warts apparently seldom occur except at the site of a callus.

Plantar warts are extremely sensitive to pressure and cause acute local discomfort. Objectively, the presence of a soft bleeding core when the overlying horny thickening has been removed, differentiates a wart from a callosity or a corn.

TREATMENT

Treatment consists in the removal of the horny callous plate or surface with a sharp safety-razor blade and cauterizing the soft center or core with acid or an electric needle. Fuming nitric, glacial acetic, or chromic acid may be used for cauterizing. Acid is applied with a sharp-pointed applicator forced deep into the core. Cauterization should be repeated every five to six days until the lesion is completely destroyed; it is necessary to remove the horny callus each time the area is cauterized. If the electric needle or electrocoagulation is used, the needle with a medium spark is thrust gently into the core of the wart. Usually, two or three applications at five to six day intervals are sufficient. Freezing with carbon dioxide snow, x-ray radiation, and radium may be used, but these have not proved as satisfactory as cauterization. If the lesion is large, surgical excision is necessary.

Since plantar warts are usually associated with callosities which indicate faulty foot balance, an important part of the treatment is overcoming this faulty foot balance. Supports designed to correct the postural faults should be provided; as plantar warts are usually found in callous areas over the metatarsal heads, a support sufficiently high and designed to protect the metatarsal heads from pressure is indicated.

RINGWORM OF THE FOOT

(Athlete's Foot)

Athlete's foot, or interdigital ringworm of the foot, is a fungus affection resulting in scales, scabs, or cracks in the webs of the toes. The organism most often found is the trichophyton fungus. Ringworm is contracted by contact with infected objects, such as shower bath mats, floors, and bath towels. It is most prevalent in young individuals and especially those engaged in sports, hence the name "Athlete's Foot."

The lesion usually appears as a very inconspicuous irritation between the toes; the only subjective symptom is burning and itching. The cracks and vesicles often become secondarily infected, and the condition assumes a true inflammatory character and tends to spread over the foot (Fig. 165). When this occurs, the foot becomes painful, inflamed, and comfortable use is interfered with.

TREATMENT

If the case is seen in its early stage when it is a true fungus infection, the treatment is rather simple and the results gratifying. Proper foot hygiene with frequent changing of hose and shoes, but with infrequent bathing of the feet and thorough drying between the toes, is the first essential in treatment. A 2 per cent solution of picric acid in 50 per cent alcohol into which a few drops of glycerine have been added, applied morning and

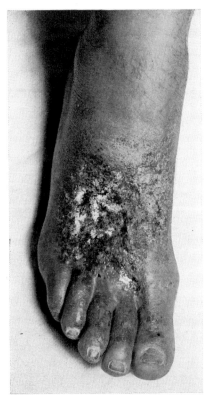

Fig. 165. Extensive "Athlete's Foot" infection. It was necessary to use x-ray to clean up this infection.

evening will usually clear up the condition. When the lesions have reached the vesicular stage with its secondary infection, bed rest is necessary, and wet compresses of a saturated solution of boric acid or 1/4000 potassium permanganate should be applied to the affected areas. The toes should be packed apart with cotton pledgets soaked in one of the above solutions. In the more persistent forms, x-ray therapy will often shorten the course of the infection but should be used in conjunction with foot hygiene.

ECZEMA

Eczema is a term commonly applied to any moist or scaly inflammation of the skin of the foot of unknown origin. It usually appears on the sides of the toes and soles of the feet and is often associated with hyperidrosis. The condition is characterized by an erythema with small papule or vesicle formation, which is accompanied by severe itching.

TREATMENT

Any source of irritation should be removed. A 5 per cent aqueous solution of silver nitrate applied three times a week will often suffice to clear up the condition. The toes should be separated by small pledgets of cotton. In persistent cases, x-ray therapy may be of value. Investigation for any general condition, dietary or otherwise, which may be responsible for the eczema, should be carried out.

HYPERIDROSIS

Hyperidrosis, more commonly known as excessive sweating of the feet, is a most disagreeable and uncomfortable affection. The condition is due to a functional disease of the sweat glands, the cause of which is unknown but is probably nervous in origin. The condition is often associated with faulty foot balance which probably acts as a contributing causative factor. Associated bacterial growths frequently complicate the condition, resulting in a very disagreeable odor. The condition is most prevalent in males.

TREATMENT

In mild cases, the frequent changing of shoes and stockings and dusting with a powder of equal parts of boric acid, salicylic acid and powdered alum at each change of footwear will usually give relief. The feet should be bathed night and morning in warm water in which an ounce of the above-mentioned dusting powder has been dissolved. In cases where the odor is particularly offensive, one of the following may be of service:

1. Bathing the feet biweekly in a foot wash of chromic acid, 40 grains to the ounce of water.
2. Wash the feet and dry thoroughly. Then paint with Commercial Formalin, 40%, ten parts, water 90 parts. Allow this to dry on the feet and repeat daily.
3. Feet may be soaked daily in 1 to 1000 solution of potassium permanganate.

Any general etiologic factors should be corrected.

14

AFFECTIONS OF THE TARSAL AND METATARSAL BONES

KÖHLER'S DISEASE OF THE TARSAL SCAPHOID

Köhler's disease is an uncommon affection of the tarsal scaphoid which causes local discomfort and tends toward spontaneous healing. Köhler's disease occurs in young children between the ages of four and seven years and is found more frequently in boys than in girls.

ETIOLOGY

The etiology of this condition is not clearly established, but it probably lies in a group of degenerative bone conditions which occur in the young, usually considered to be caused by interference with the local circulation or low-grade infection. Trauma undoubtedly is a contributing causative factor; such trauma may be an acute injury or may take the form of a repeated insult due to faulty foot balance with concentration of weight stresses on the scaphoid bone.

PATHOLOGY

Necrotic changes in the cancellous bone with replacement fibrosis has been found in microscopic sections.

SYMPTOMS

Localized pain over the scaphoid bone, aggravated by use, and limp are the most common subjective symptoms. Objectively, there is tenderness over the scaphoid bone and, at times, swelling. X-ray plates taken in the dorsiplantar and lateral planes show a very characteristic picture; the tarsal scaphoid is small, dense, often irregular, and narrow in its anterior-posterior diameter (Fig. 166).

TREATMENT

In the acute stage of the disease, complete rest in a plaster cast is necessary; the cast should be worn for several weeks or until the acute symptoms have subsided. After removal of the cast, a support should be used to protect the scaphoid bone from weight

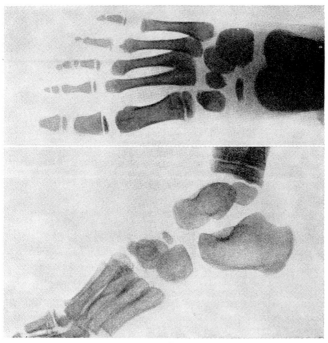

FIG. 166. Köhler's disease of the tarsal scaphoid. Note thinning and condensation of the scaphoid bone.

stresses and correct faulty foot posture. A stout, well-designed shoe should be worn. Foci of infection should be sought for and eliminated if found. The administration of calcium and cod-liver oil is also indicated to hasten healing and recalcification of the decalcified bone areas.

MARCH FOOT

March foot is a condition characterized by a painful swelling on the dorsum of the forefoot, often associated with a spontaneous fracture of one of the metatarsal bones, usually the second or third (Fig. 167).

ETIOLOGY

March foot was first described by Briehaupt in 1855. Briehaupt observed a malady which occurred in German soldiers after pro-

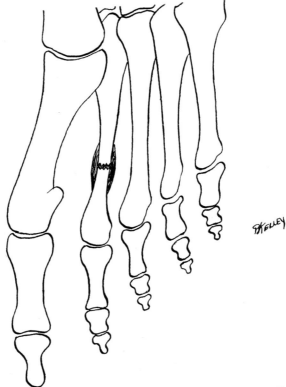

FIG. 167. Schematic drawing of a march-foot fracture with excess callus formation.

longed marching, described as a "persistent, edematous and painful foot." The association of spontaneous fracture of the metatarsal bone was not described by Briehaupt. Later, in 1877, the French military surgeon, Pauzet, described a similar condition; he considered it to be a periosteal irritation of the metatarsal bones. Deutschander, in 1921, was the first to describe the condition in the civilian. Excessive use of the foot, such as long marches or prolonged walking in civilian life, is unquestionably an exciting cause of march foot. Faulty foot balance with concentration of weight stresses on the second, third or fourth metatarsal bones seems to be an important contributing factor as many of the reported cases had a previous history of some form of functional foot disorder. Interference with the blood supply

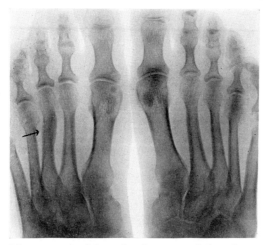

Fig. 168. Dorsiplantar x-ray of foot showing a march-foot fracture of the third metatarsal bone.

with weakening of the bones has been suggested as a cause of march foot, as has also spasm of the interosseus muscle. It seems probable, however, that extensive use of the forepart of the foot under adverse conditions is the most logical explanation of the condition.

PATHOLOGY

In the early stages of march foot and in arrested cases, there is no discernible pathology. When spontaneous fracture occurs, there is periosteal proliferation, fracture of the involved metatarsal bone, and finally, as healing progresses, excess callus formation (Fig. 168).

Symptoms

Subjectively, pain is complained of in the forefoot which gradually increases until walking is seriously interfered with or is impossible. Objectively, there is swelling over the dorsum of the foot with localized redness and pain. There is an area tender to pressure over the distal part of the second or third metatarsal bone. If fracture is present, it is impossible to bear weight on the foot. X-ray evidence of any pathology is often lacking for the first week or two after the onset of the pain. After the lapse of a week or two, an x-ray will show a periosteal fuzziness at the site of the beginning fracture. Careful inspection may show a trace of a fracture line at this time. A little later the periosteal shadow becomes more distinct and the fracture line is plainly evident. At times, perhaps more frequently than otherwise, no definite fracture line can be seen, and only an actively proliferating mass of callus is discernible. Fracture of more than one metatarsal is rare.

Treatment

Recognition of the prodromal symptoms before fracture occurs is important. In this stage, relief from weight-bearing and local heat and support will usually arrest the condition, and in two to three weeks the foot will return to normal. After fracture has occurred, immobilization in a plaster cast or by strapping should be used for two to three weeks. When weight-bearing is resumed, the foot should be carefully balanced to overcome any postural defects which may be present. Support for the metatarsal and longitudinal arches is indicated even if no obvious faulty balance is present; such support protects the fractured area and makes walking and weight-bearing much more comfortable. Supports should be continued for some weeks after walking has been resumed.

INFRACTION OF THE SECOND METATARSAL BONE
(Freiberg's Disease)

Freiberg, Köhler, and others have described an affection of the head of the second metatarsal bone characterized by degenerative changes in the head of the bone with painful symptoms in the metatarsophalangeal joint of the second toe. This condition occurs almost exclusively in the adolescent period.

ETIOLOGY

The etiology of this condition is by no means clear, but it is believed to be caused by some interference with circulation which results in an aseptic necrosis of the head of the bone. Our observations in a comparatively few cases have led us to believe that a short first metatarsal bone with concentration of weight on the head of the second metatarsal bone may have some bearing on the causation of this condition. Such a faulty structural arrangement exposes the head of the second metatarsal to trauma, either accidental or from ordinary use. Trauma unquestionably plays a contributing role in the causation of the condition.

PATHOLOGY

There are degenerative changes in the head of the second metatarsal bone, which becomes distorted and irregular. Köhler calls attention to a thickening of the shaft of the second metatarsal as a part of the morbid process (Fig. 169). It is interesting in this connection to note that with a short first metatarsal bone, thickening of the shaft of the second metatarsal is nearly always observed; this would seem to indicate that a short first metatarsal may be of some importance as a causative factor in the production of infraction of the second metatarsal head.

SYMPTOMS

Pain is complained of over the head of the second metatarsal bone on weight-bearing, and walking is interfered with. Objectively, there is localized swelling and thickening of the metatarsophalangeal joint of the second toe. The joint is usually quite tender to pressure, and may show evidence of inflammatory reaction. X-rays taken in the dorsiplantar plane show characteristic changes in the head of the second metatarsal bone. The metatarsal head is flattened, it is broadened in the neck, and the whole shaft of the bone is thicker and denser than normal. The joint space is widened and loose bodies may be present; when the epiphyseal line is visible, it is very irregular (Fig. 170). The base of the proximal phalanx displays similar changes in a lesser degree. In old and advanced cases, the appearance of the joint is very decidedly that of an extensive osteo-arthritis.

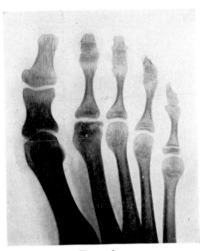 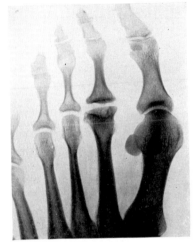

FIG. 169   FIG. 170

FIG. 169. Infraction of the head of metatarsal II; note the hypertrophy of metatarsal II.

FIG. 170. Infraction of the head of the second metatarsal. Case of long standing with distortion of the metatarsophalangeal joint.

TREATMENT

The treatment consists of complete immobilization in a plaster cast if the condition is acute and painful. Following such a period of complete immobilization, the foot should be carefully balanced to overcome any postural faults present, and adequate support should be placed under the metatarsal arch to prevent the head of the second metatarsal from bearing weight. Such conservative treatment, if persisted in, will usually bring about subsidence of acute symptoms, but the joint must be protected for a long period of time from weight-bearing by the use of a metatarsal support (Fig. 171). Occasionally, particularly in the older cases, remodeling or a complete resection of the malformed head of the second metatarsal may be necessary for relief. Following such

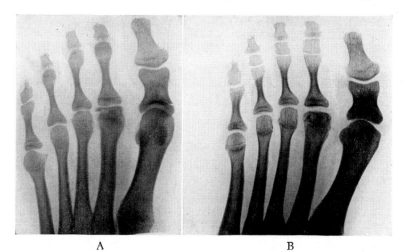

A   B

Fig. 171. Infraction of the head of metatarsal II. A, before treatment; B, after several months of treatment.

operative correction, the continued use of a support for the meta-tarsal arch is necessary.

15

AFFECTIONS OF THE HEEL

Painful and sensitive areas about the heel are not uncommon, and give rise to considerable discomfort. Such painful points are caused by inflammation or irritation of tendon sheaths and bursae or a periostitis with proliferative changes, involving the posterior and inferior surfaces of the os calcis. The most common painful heel conditions are the following:

CALCANEAL SPURS

Proliferative changes occur over the tuberosity of the os calcis at the attachment of the plantar fascia which frequently develop

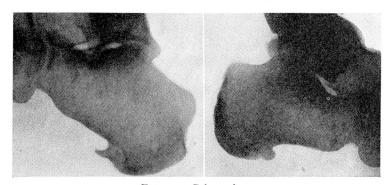

Fig. 172. Calcaneal spurs.

into spurs or spur-like prominences (Fig. 172). Formerly, calcaneal spurs were considered to be always caused by a Neisserian infection, but any type of systemic infection may be responsible for their development. In addition to systemic infection, local irritation caused by faulty foot attitude, or acute or repeated trauma, is an important factor. A small adventitious bursa sometimes covers the calcaneal spur and a definite bursitis may develop in this bursa.

Symptoms

Pain in the heel over the tuberosity of the os calcis aggravated by weight-bearing is the most important subjective complaint.

Objectively, there is a definite point of acute tenderness over the tuberosity of the os calcis, and frequently a bony projection can be palpated at this point. A lateral x-ray will show proliferative changes over the tuberosity of the os calcis and frequently, but not always, a true spur formation.

TREATMENT

Conservative treatment will, as a rule, give relief. The painful symptoms complained of are due to bursitis or periosteal irrita-

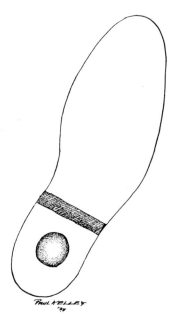

FIG. 173. Shape, contour, and placement of sponge-rubber heel pad to relieve pressure on the calcaneal spur.

tion rather than the presence of a bony outgrowth in the majority of cases, and if adequate protection is given the irritated area, the acute reaction will quiet down and pain will disappear. Complete rest and the use of hot applications are indicated when the condition is acute and very painful. After the subsidence of the acute symptoms and in mild cases, the shoe should be balanced to relieve the painful area from weight-bearing. The most usual device employed for this purpose is a soft pad made of sponge

rubber with a hole or hollow in its center into which the tuberosity of the os calcis fits (Fig. 173). A more satisfactory device is
a bar of sponge rubber placed across the insole of the shoe just
anterior to the painful point (Fig. 174). This bar is one-fourth
to one-half inch thick, one and one-half inches broad, and tapers
gradually anteriorly and rather abruptly posteriorly. Such a cal-

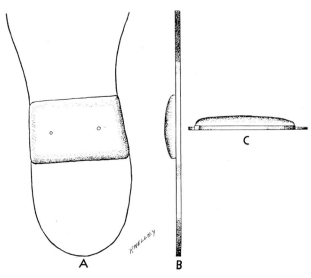

FIG. 174. Sponge-rubber calcaneal bar used in treatment of painful heels. A, shape
and placement of bar in shoe; B, contour, side view; C, contour, anterior view.

caneal bar effectively relieves the painful areas from pressure in
weight-bearing and is quite comfortable. A sponge-rubber inlay
which concentrates weight on the forepart of the foot and relieves the heel of the weight-bearing stress may be used advantageously in conjunction with a calcaneal bar; this combination
will often give relief if the bar alone fails (Fig. 175).

Injection Treatment. Since, as a rule, pain over a calcaneal
spur is due to irritation caused by a calcareous deposit at the point
where the plantar fascia inserts into the spur, or to inflammation
of a small adventitious bursa, occasionally found at the tip of the
spur, injection of the painful area will at times give rapid relief.
Eucipin procaine is most commonly used for this purpose, about

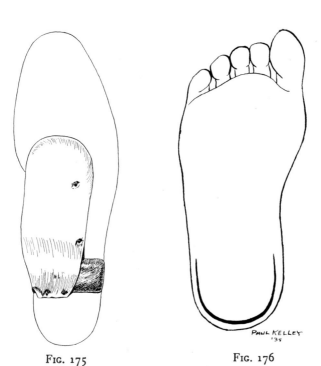

FIG. 175   FIG. 176

FIG. 175. Calcaneal bar as used in combination with support. Shape and placement of bar and support in shoe.
FIG. 176. Incision used for removal of calcaneal spurs.

5 cc. being infiltrated into the painful area. Two or thre
will usually determine whether this form of treatme
effective. The patient should be warned, however, tha
may become extremely painful within a few hours afte
and may remain so for twelve to twenty-four hours.
treatment should be used in conjunction with the protect
ures which have already been described.

Occasionally, when there is definite spur formation, p
sensitiveness in the heel persist in spite of all conservativ
ures, and removal of the spur by operation is necessar
incision used is a U-shaped one around the heel, parallel
just above the sole (Fig. 176). A flap composed of skin a
is turned back, and the tuberosity of the os calcis is fully exposed.
The spur, with a thin slice of cortical bone, is excised from the
under surface of the os calcis and the flap is sutured back into
place. Following operation, provision should be made to protect
the heel from weight-bearing for some weeks. Removal of calcaneal
spurs by operation is not always a success so far as relief from
symptoms is concerned, and it is advisable to avoid operative interference if possible.

CALCANEAL APOPHYSITIS

(Epiphysitis of the Os Calcis)

The os calcis is the only tarsal bone which always has an epiphysis. This epiphysis, which lies at the tip of the heel and re-
ceives the attachment of the tendo achillis, consequently may be
partially separated in childhood by excessive strain exerted through
the heel tendon and symptoms develop which resemble apophysitis. Apophysitis, however, is a different condition and represents
a true degenerative affection involving the epiphysis. It occurs
most often in boys between the ages of ten and fifteen years
(Fig. 177).

ETIOLOGY

The etiology of apophysitis is still unsettled; the following are the most commonly accepted etiological factors: (1) direct trauma or strain from the attachment of the powerful heel tendon; (2) circulatory or nutritional disturbances of the epiphysis, prob-

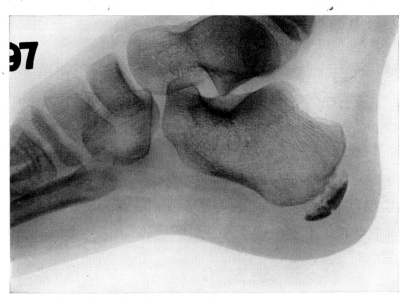

FIG. 177. X-ray of os calcis showing irregular epiphysis and fragmentation-calcaneal apophysitis.

ably secondary to trauma; (3) systemic infections; (4) endocrine imbalance, usually hypopituitarism. The condition of apophysitis is undoubtedly analogous in origin, etiology, and pathology with such epiphyseal disturbances as Legg's disease in the head of the femur; Osgood Schlatter's disease of the tibia; Frieberg's disease of the second metatarsal head; and Köhler's disease in the tarsal scaphoid.

SYMPTOMS

The onset of apophysitis is generally gradual and insidious. The first symptom is usually a slight limp which is followed by definite pain localized on the posterior aspect of the os calcis at the tip of the heel. An area of tenderness over the tip of the heel may be elicited by the lateral palpation of the heel with the index finger and thumb. Usually, the line of tenderness to pressure follows the outline of the calcaneal epiphysis. There is, at times, some swelling of the lateral and medial aspects of the heel and, in cases of long standing, edema may be present. An x-ray taken in the lateral plane will show the epiphysis to be irregular and segmented with areas of increased density (Fig. 177).

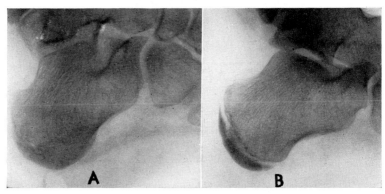

Fig. 178. Calcaneal apophysitis. A, acute stage of the infection (note the loss of demarcation of epiphyseal line); B, same case several months after treatment.

Treatment

If the condition is treated in its acute stage, it can, as a rule, be rapidly terminated. Treatment should consist of complete rest of the involved foot secured by the application of a plaster cast from above the knee to the ends of the toes; this cast prevents tension on the heel cord and should be worn two to three weeks. At the end of this time, a light cast extending from below the knee to the toes should be applied and worn for another two to three weeks. After the removal of such cast, if the painful symptoms have subsided, a strapping of adhesive should be applied about the heel and ankle to limit the pull of the tendo achillis. The shoe should be padded to relieve the heel from weight-bearing for several months. This is accomplished by the use of a rubber heel pad or calcaneal bar. Faulty foot attitude should be corrected by adequate supports and shoe alterations. The administration of calcium and cod-liver oil is, at times, indicated, and if there is evidence of endocrine imbalance, this should be treated (Fig. 178).

TENOSYNOVITIS OF THE TENDO ACHILLIS

This condition is similar to a tenosynovitis involving any tendon sheath. Systemic infection and local irritation are the causative factors. The condition is characterized by local pain, swelling, and redness over the tendo achillis and crepitation over the tendon on movement. Treatment consists of rest and the local application of moist heat. In severe cases, the tendon should be completely immobilized for a week to ten days in a plaster cast, but as a rule a basket strapping will immobilize the heel and limit the movement of the heel tendon which is all that is necessary for recovery. Focal infections should be sought for and eliminated if found.

BURSITIS

The bursa most commonly involved is the retrocalcaneal bursa (Fig. 179B), which lies between the os calcis and the tendo achillis. Inflammation of this bursa is characterized by local pain, tenderness, and swelling; swelling, when present, is localized on the sides of the heel cord. Local periostitis with proliferative changes and irregular spur formation on the posterior surface of the os calcis are occasionally found associated with inflammation of this bursa and may indeed be the real cause of the bursitis (Fig. 180). Local heat and rest are the mainstays in treatment but at times complete immobilization of the ankle joint in a plaster cast is indicated. Strapping with adhesive is also of service. Sources of focal infection should be searched for and eradicated. If the bursitis does not subside under conservative measures, the bursa should be excised. When the retrocalcaneal bursa is excised, it must be completely removed; this may require considerable dissection, as the bursa is often surprisingly extensive and may have several off-

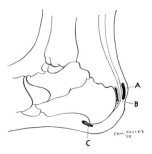

FIG. 179. Bursae of the heel. A, posterior achilles; B, retrocalcaneal; C, inferior calcaneal bursae.

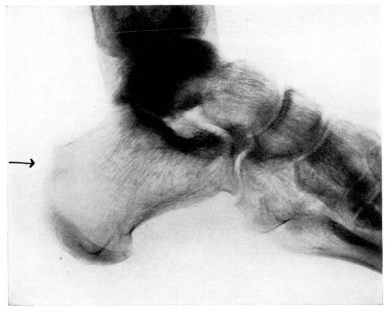

FIG. 180. Calcaneobursitis. Note the moth-eaten appearance on the posterior sur-face of the os calcis, beneath the bursa.

shoots or pockets which must be traced down and dissected out. When hypertrophic spurs are present, they must be carefully and completely removed.

Friction of the heel counter of the shoe may cause a bursitis of the superficial calcaneal (posterior achillis) bursa which lies between the heel tendon and the skin (Fig. 179A). Such a superficial bursitis can usually be relieved by the application of heat and protecting the area by an adhesive strapping. This condition is at times associated with faulty foot attitude and this should always be corrected. At times the bursa must be excised. It should never be incised.

16

FUNCTIONAL DISORDERS OF THE FOOT IN RELATION TO MILITARY SERVICE

The sedentary habits which have become so prevalent in this country because of widespread transportation facilities and the increased introduction of machinery in our manufacturing plants have tended to bring about such a decided national weakness of the feet that the strain incidental to strenuous military duty can cause considerable disability. The correct appraisal of the foot of the inductee and the care of the soldier's feet after his induction have become, then, matters of considerable importance.

It is generally recognized that the efficiency of a fighting unit depends upon the physical fitness of its personnel. Included in physical fitness is a pair of sound feet, capable of standing up under the demands made upon them. Only strong feet can stand the strain and stress of strenuous military training, and it is not surprising that symptom-free but potentially weak feet break down when subjected to long marches, under full equipment. It follows that in the selection of men for military service, if the unfit are to be eliminated and those with potential foot weaknesses properly classified, the capacity of the foot must be appraised in relation to what will be required of it. Likewise, we must recognize and treat in their incipience the various minor affections which will occur among those accepted and so prevent complete foot breakdown, for even with careful selection and proper fitting with regulation shoes, a great deal of foot trouble will develop and has developed on active duty, and that in spite of apparently adequate feet.

APPRAISAL OF A FOOT FOR MILITARY SERVICE

In arriving at a decision as to the fitness of a selectee for active duty, the general make-up of the individual as well as the condition of the foot must be taken into consideration.

General Factors Worthy of Consideration. The general make-up of the individual is often significant. A short, stocky individual is not often subject to foot strain; the tall, slender, visceroptotic type, with long, slender, flexible feet, on the other hand, is often subject to foot strain under continued and unaccustomed use. If, to a relaxed general make-up, are added poor posture with a sway back, protuberant abdomen, and round shoulders, the individual is not likely to stand up well under the strain of the strenuous activity of a combat unit, and probably foot strain will be the first indication of a breakdown.

Knock Knee, Bow Leg, and Tibial Torsion. Knock knee, bow leg, and tibial torsion tend to cause foot strain. Normally, the line of transmitted weight passes approximately through the middle of the patella and falls between metatarsals I and II. Knock knee, bow leg, and tibial torsion cause a shift of the line of transmitted weight, so that weight stresses fall upon the foot in an abnormal manner. This shift of weight is toward the medial side of the foot, so that the weight-bearing thrust is concentrated on metatarsal I, or internal to it (Fig. 96). Concentration of weight stresses on the medial side of the foot rolls the foot downward and inward, throws the os calcis into a valgus position, and inevitably results in pronation. Of these three conditions, bow leg is the least likely to cause trouble in the young and more vigorous groups, particularly since it is usually found in the stocky type of individual; in the older age groups, bow leg quite frequently leads to foot and knee strain. These postural defects should be given consideration in estimating the physical endurance of the selectee.

EXAMINATION OF THE FOOT

When the foot itself is examined, it should be carefully inspected with the shoe on. Bulging of either the inner or the outer side of the shoe, especially wearing down the inner side of the heel and sole, suggests faulty foot balance. A turned-up sole and a hole in the ball of the shoe suggest a depressed anterior arch.

With the shoes removed, the posture of the foot should be carefully estimated and departures from the normal searched for; some of these latter may be trivial and readily corrected, whereas others make anything but limited duty impossible.

Pronation or inward rolling of the foot is a very definite indication of a weak foot. In all pronated feet, the scaphoid bone and the internal malleolus are prominent when the foot is viewed from the front. When viewed from behind with the feet parallel, the os calcis or heel bone will be found to be in a very definitely valgus position (Fig. 73). The height of the long arch is much less important than the presence of pronation as an indication of weak feet, since the height of the arch shows wide variation in different individuals; many low-arched or flatfeet are perfectly sound and capable of strenuous use, always provided pronation is not present in addition. A man should not be turned down for active duty because of the presence of a low arch alone.

Arthritic Flatfoot. This descriptive term is applied to a foot which is pronated, flat, and with limited or complete loss of movement in all or most of the foot joints. The underlying cause of this condition is focal infection, but faulty foot attitude is usually associated. An arthritic flatfoot with limited foot-joint motion should be considered a cause for rejection for military service.

A high-arched foot (Fig. 116) is usually associated with prominent ball and contracted toes. A high-arched foot in younger individuals is a quite serviceable foot but becomes less adaptable to strenuous use as the age of forty or forty-five is approached. The high-arched foot with hammertoes and prominent ball, covered with a heavy callus, is a type of foot which will not stand excessive use and strain and should be classified as a potentially weak foot, at least in those over thirty-five years of age.

Hammertoe deformity (Fig. 154) is characterized by contractures of the midphalangeal joint in acute flexion. Usually this joint is covered by callus or corn. When the hammertoe is flexible —that is, when there is no ankylosis of the joint—it can cause little trouble, but when it is rigid and covered by heavy callus, the hammertoe is painful when pressed upon by the shoe. Hammertoe alone does not demand rejection, since it is readily corrected by a comparatively slight operation.

Hallux valgus, or bunions (Fig. 139) is characterized by enlargement of the great toe joint and deviation of the great toe toward the lateral or outer side of the foot. If mild, this condition is not a cause for rejection. If there is marked valgus or outward deviation of the great toe present, however, the individual should be rejected, for even if the deformity is corrected by operation, the soldier practically never resumes full active duty.

Tailor's bunion, or enlargement of the tuberosity of the fifth metatarsal bone, on the outer side of the foot, can cause considerable foot disability. It is characterized by swelling, tenderness, and redness on the lateral surface of the foot, just posterior to the fifth toe. This condition is readily corrected by a simple operation, and should not be considered a cause for rejection.

Rigid toe is a painful condition, involving the metatarsophalangeal joint of the great toe. The condition is characterized by limitation of motion in the great toe joint, usually in the direction of dorsal flexion, and pain in the joint following walking, particularly on uneven ground. Hallux rigidus is always a cause for rejection. Here again, even if the condition is corrected by operation, a range of motion permitting extensive use of the foot is seldom restored, particularly in marching.

Calcaneal Bursitis (Fig. 179). This condition is characterized by redness, tenderness, and swelling, localized over the tendo achillis at its insertion into the os calcis. Calcaneal bursitis is readily irritated by friction from the heel of the shoe, but since this bursa can be removed by a simple operation, it should not be considered a reason for rejection.

Spastic Flatfoot. The tone and general development of the muscles in the foot and leg should be carefully investigated. This is best done by watching active movements in various directions. Tautness or spasticity of the peroneal muscles (indicated by limited ability to adduct the foot or roll it inward), and shortness of the heel tendon (indicated by the individual's inability to dorsally flex the foot in adduction to a right angle or better), are common causes of foot breakdown, and the resulting condition is sometimes referred to as "spastic flatfoot." Shortening and spasticity of these muscle groups, however, usually can be overcome by carefully planned exercises, and should not be considered causes for rejection.

Spurs on the Os Calcis. Pain on the plantar surface of the heel is caused by enlargement of the tuberosity of the os calcis, which may be so extensive as to form a spur, often readily palpable and always demonstrable by x-ray. This condition is characterized by an area of pain and tenderness always localized over the tuberosity of the os calcis and discomfort or acute pain on weight-bearing in the same area. A true spur formation demonstrable by x-ray demands rejection, for such a foot always breaks down under extensive use and becomes extremely painful.

X-ray examination, especially views taken in the weight-bearing position, are helpful in evaluating the condition of the foot, particularly those showing evidences of departure from the normal. It must be confessed, however, that foot x-rays are not particularly enlightening except to one who has had considerable experience in interpreting them.

These are the most common conditions found in the foot which give rise to functional foot disorders and thereby (1) prevent military service, (2) require correction if active duty is to be expected, or (3) call for classification for limited duty.

PHYSICAL STANDARDS FOR THE FEET*

Acceptable Conditions for Class 1 A

Pes planus, unless accompanied by marked deformity, rigidity, or weakness, or of such degree as to have interfered with useful vocation in civil life.

Hallux valgus, unless severe.

Clubfoot, of slight degree, if tarsal, metatarsal, and phalangeal joints are flexible and the condition permits the wearing of a military shoe and, in the opinion of the examiner, will not interfere with the performance of military duty.

Slight claw toes, not involving obliteration of the transverse arch, which do not interfere with the wearing of a military shoe.

Hammertoe, which is flexible and which does not interfere with the wearing of a military shoe. (Hammertoe usually involves the second digit, and, unless it is rigid, is not a disqualifying defect.)

* United States Selective Service Regulations, October 18, 1940.

Absence of one or two of the small toes, of one or both feet, if the function of the foot is good.

Ingrowing toe nails.

Acceptable Conditions for Class 1 B

Abduction and pronation (knock-ankle) when this condition is not associated with rigidity of the tarsal joint or with deformity of the foot. (This defect is remediable with proper foot exercises and with correct shoes.)

Loss of great toe.

Loss of dorsal flexion of the great toe.

Hammertoe, with rigidity.

Other defects of the feet which disqualify for general military service, but which do not prevent the registrant from wearing a military shoe and which have not prevented him from following a useful vocation in civil life.

Conditions Which Warrant Rejection (Class 4)

Pes planus, if accompanied by marked deformity, rigidity, or weakness, or of such degree as to have interfered with useful vocation in civil life.

Obliteration of the transverse arch, associated with permanent flexion of the small toes (claw toes).

Hallux valgus, if severe and associated with marked exostosis or bunion, especially when there are signs of irritation above the joint.

Clubfoot, if marked in degree, or which interferes with the wearing of a military shoe.

Amputations of extremities in excess of those already cited.

SERVICE-INDUCED FOOT DISORDERS

It may be taken for granted that of the men inducted into the service, some will have excellent feet, able to withstand any amount of work. Some will have structurally normal feet, but feet which are potentially weak because of the sedentary life which has been led; in this group, as a consequence of lack of healthy use, the ligaments are weak, and important muscles are below par in strength and development. Some will have minor foot defects insufficient to cause symptoms in civil life, but which can become disabling under the stress of military activity. It is the latter two groups which are likely to cause loss of man power, interfering with smooth functioning of active military units.

The man with strong feet needs little discussion. The observation of commonsense rules of foot hygiene—that is, bathing the feet daily (or more often if extensive marching is engaged in), changing the hose frequently enough to insure that dirty, sweaty foot coverings do not cause irritation and blisters, and fitting the foot with a shoe of the proper size (page 212), are all that is needed to keep such a foot in good condition.

Effects of a Sedentary Life. The man with the well-balanced foot which, however, has never been called upon to meet the strain of extensive use will present a real opportunity for prophylactic care. It should be the duty of every medical officer attached to troops to know the physical, and, if possible, the mental make-up of the men for whose health he is responsible. An intelligent and energetic medical officer will give careful attention to his men's feet and should, after a little experience aided by readily obtainable information, be able fairly accurately to appraise the feet of those in his command and prevent foot breakdown.

This group we are discussing needs intelligent preliminary training directed toward toughening up the ligaments and gradually developing and strengthening the leg and foot muscles, before they can successfully withstand the strain of unaccustomed activity. By following thoughtfully worked-out plans designed to provide gradually toughening-up training, such feet can, within two to four weeks, be put in condition to stand up on hikes of reasonable length, and from this point rapidly progress to long hikes with full equipment.

The wide-awake medical officer will segregate this group from the group with strong feet, put them on exercises (page 330), have them engage in athletic games of which a large variety can be devised, and carry out hikes over gradually increasing distances. Such a régime together with instruction in foot hygiene will rapidly convert this group from potential foot casualties into a group capable of carrying on efficiently. It is true that malingering must be constantly guarded against, but this is not a difficult problem if the feet are periodically examined and checked over.

Men with Minor Foot Defects. The third group constitutes a real problem. Hammertoes become irritated and painful, mild bunions or tailor's bunions become swollen and inflamed, calcaneal bursitis makes marching almost impossible, and acute foot strain practically incapacitates. Of these conditions, acute foot strain requires only intelligent management. Hammertoe, tailor's bunion, and calcaneal bursitis require hospitalization and the operative removal of the cause, as these conditions can safely be operated upon and the man returned to duty. Bunions or hallux valgus, calcaneal spurs, and rigid first toes practically never can be operated upon and the soldier returned to duty, and operations on these conditions should not be advised in military service.

TREATMENT OF COMMON FOOT CONDITIONS INCIDENT TO MILITARY SERVICE

Acute Foot Strain

This condition occurs when the work that the foot is called upon to perform is greater than its capacity. The symptoms vary from complaints of foot tire to severe pain in the long arch of the foot often associated with pain in the calf of the leg and in the knees. Objectively, the foot may be slightly swollen, and there may be tender spots in the sole, over the scaphoid-astragalar joint (Fig. 71) and plantar fascia; not uncommonly cramps in the calf of the legs are complained of.

Treatment. Treatment consists in complete bed rest until all acute symptoms subside. Attempts to cure an acute foot strain by partial rest and part-time duty with supporting strapping serves only to prolong convalescence and usually fails to correct the condition. Contrast baths and exercises carried out without weight-bearing are helpful and should be a part of the treatment. As soon as weight-bearing is pain-free, foot exercises should be prescribed and religiously carried out. Such a régime will usually restore the soldier to full duty in a reasonable length of time and keep him on full duty, provided there is no serious foot imbalance present.

Metatarsal Pain (Metatarsalgia)

Not infrequently, foot strain manifests itself as a painful condition of the metatarsal arch in the fore part of the foot. Metatarsalgia is at times associated with strain of the longitudinal arch but is more common in the high-arched foot with its prominent ball, which is frequently covered by a thick, hard callus.

Treatment. Metatarsalgia requires complete bed rest until the acute symptoms subside, though usually the rest period is not so prolonged as that in strain of the longitudinal arch. In cases in which a prominent ball is covered with callus, or there is definite weakness or descent of the metatarsal arch, the shoe should be balanced in a manner described below.

While, in civil life, arch supports can be very satisfactorily used to relieve foot strain, their use does not seem to have any place in military service except for those in the less active branches or on limited duty. It is quite possible, however, by altering the balance of the shoe, by making certain minor adjustments in the sole, to protect a mildly unbalanced foot and make it capable of carrying on quite satisfactorily.

In a mildly pronated foot in which the os calcis tends to assume a position of valgus, the condition can be materially improved by wedging the inner side of the heel of the shoe one-eighth to three-sixteenths inch and placing a wedge one-eighth inch thick in the outer side of the sole of the shoe opposite the head of the fifth metatarsal bone (Figs. 113-114). Altering the balance of the sole of the shoe in this way tends to roll the os calcis into a varus position and correct mild pronation; the wedge in the outer side of the shoe prevents the foot from sliding outward when the heel is elevated on the inside. Extending the inner side of the heel forward (Thomas heel, Fig. 115) acts in very much the same way and may be used. With pain in the metatarsal arch and callus formation on the bottom of the foot, the metatarsal arch can be relieved of weight-bearing by placing a bar of leather across the sole of the shoe just posterior to the head of the metatarsal bones (Fig. 123).

Such simple shoe alterations can readily be made, are quite

helpful, and should be utilized to keep on duty men who otherwise would become incapacitated.

IRRITATED AND RIGID HAMMERTOES

Men suffering from this condition should be hospitalized and the toe deformity corrected by operation. (See page 247.)

CALCANEAL BURSITIS

This condition may respond to conservative treatment, and so, if it is mild, strapping of the area to protect it from friction may be successful. If this simple conservative measure fails, the patient should be hospitalized and complete excision of the bursa and the underlying rough bone should be carried out. (See page 283.)

INGROWING TOE NAILS

Ingrowing toe nails can become a very incapacitating condition, particularly the type with a mild superimposed infection. Proper shoeing and trimming the nails straight across instead of rounding the corners and packing under the corner of the nail with a slight film of cotton will take care of the mild case of ingrowing toe nail (Fig. 158). If the condition fails to respond to conservative treatment, hospitalization and a properly performed operation will remove the cause and return the man to duty (page 254). Removal of the nail is not a cure for ingrowing toe nail, and usually results in an abnormal nail which continues to be troublesome. Removal of half of the nail is even less successful. Unless the operation is to be performed correctly, it had better not be done.

PLANTAR WARTS

Plantar warts are small, circumscribed callus-like growths which form on the plantar surface of the foot and heel. They are often confused with callosities and corns. If the horny top of the plantar wart is removed with a razor blade, a soft central core which is exquisitely tender and bleeds readily will be found. Such plantar warts are very painful and make weight-bearing at times almost impossible.

Treatment consists in removing the horny callous surface with a razor blade and thoroughly cauterizing the center or core with fuming nitric acid or an electric needle if that is available. The acid should be applied on a sharp, pointed applicator, and should be forced deeply into the core until it penetrates into the underlying subcutaneous tissue. Usually a drop of blood will ooze out. If the plantar wart is small, one treatment of nitric acid will usually cure the condition. If the wart is of long duration and is large, a number of treatments will be necessary. These should then be repeated at weekly intervals, care being taken at each application to shave off the horny covering before the soft underlying part is cauterized.

Athlete's Foot

Athlete's foot is a fungus infection, resulting in scales, scabs, or cracks in the webs of the toes. The organism most often found is a trichophyton fungus. Athlete's foot is contracted by contact with infected objects, such as showerbath mats, floors, and bath towels. The lesion usually appears as a very inconspicuous irritation between the toes, the only subjective symptoms being burning and itching. The cracks and vesicles often become secondarily infected, and the condition assumes a true inflammatory character and tends to spread over the foot (Fig. 165). When this occurs, the foot becomes painful and inflamed, and comfortable use is interfered with.

Treatment consists in proper foot hygiene, frequent changes of hose and shoes, but infrequent bathing of the feet. The feet should be cleansed thoroughly with alcohol, particularly between the toes. A 2 per cent solution of picric acid in 50 per cent alcohol to which a few drops of glycerine have been added, applied once a day, will usually clear up the condition. In the more persistent cases, x-ray therapy will often shorten the course of the infection; x-ray should be used in conjunction with foot hygiene.

Frost-Bite or Chilblains

This condition is caused by exposure to extreme cold. The parts of the foot chiefly affected, because they have the least circulation, are the toes and the back of the heel. A high wind is a contributing cause, and lack of oxygen is an important factor in the case of aviators. Initially, there is a burning sensation in the affected part of the foot, and as this subsides the affected parts become numb. At this stage, the skin is white and the toes become stiff. The general result varies from complete recovery to ulceration, and, in severe cases, gangrene.

Treatment. Prophylactic treatment is most important; this consists in properly fitting shoes and hose and adequate clothing for the body to keep up the general circulation. The shoes should be kept well oiled and dry, and the wearing of wet or soiled socks should be avoided. In the acute stage, the application of heat should be avoided, as should rubbing. The feet should be elevated and wrapped in woolen coverings for a short period of time. Following this, the feet should not be treated with heat but should be refrigerated by placing ice packs around the foot, well protected by a woolen covering, until the natural color appears, indicating that circulation has returned to normal.

The pathology is one in which the blood supply to the involved parts has been definitely or even severely interfered with. This being the case, reducing the demand for blood supply by decreasing metabolic activity in the involved area by lowering the temperature enables the tissues to survive until the vascular spasm relaxes and the normal volume of blood gradually finds access to them. Such refrigeration will frequently prevent necrosis and gangrene. Heat, on the other hand, raises the metabolic activity in the tissues. This increased metabolic activity demands a greater blood supply which the tissues cannot receive because of the reduced caliper of the vessels, and ulceration and gangrene are favored.

TRENCH FOOT

This is a neurocirculatory disturbance caused by prolonged exposure to cold and dampness. This condition develops after standing for long periods in dampness and mud with inactive muscles. It very closely resembles frost-bite, and the symptoms are almost identical. The method of treatment is the same as that used for frost-bite; namely, proper prophylactic measures directed toward keeping the feet warm and dry. Effective treatment of the condition, once it has occurred, consists in elevation, protection, and mild refrigeration until the neurocirculatory condition has subsided and the circulation returns to normal.

IMMERSION FOOT

Immersion foot is a condition produced by long immersion in extremely cold water, usually associated with immobility of the limbs and constriction of the lower extremities by shoes, boots, or clothing. While immersion in water showing a low temperature (34 to 36° F.) has been responsible for most of the cases of immersion foot, the condition has been seen following immersion in tropical waters of a much higher temperature. A case of immersion foot has come under the authors' observation which occurred following six days in an open boat in the Caribbean (usual temperature, 60 to 70° F.). Immersion foot is similar to "trench foot" and "shelter foot."

The pathology is an intense vasodilatation with transudation of serum and blood and subsequent profound inflammatory reaction.

The symptoms vary, depending upon the severity of the condition and the time element. At the time of removal from the open boat or raft, the feet are cold and waxy white in color, with scattered cyanotic areas. Numbness and anesthesia to pain, touch, and temperature are present. Later the feet become red, hyperemic, and hot, and the pulse in the vessels of the feet is full and bounding. The toes, the distal portion of the dorsum of the foot, and ball of the foot show the greatest reaction, and in these areas blebs may form, filled with straw-colored fluid or extravasated blood. In severe cases, the feet present the appearance of incipient gangrene. Areas of anesthesia are present. In the milder forms, the areas of anesthesia extend around the margin of the foot and over the plantar aspect. In more severe cases, the anesthesia extends up over the entire dorsum of the foot and in some cases over the lower two-thirds of the leg.

Surgeon Commander T. R. Webster, Surgeon Lieutenant F. M. Woolhouse, and Surgeon Lieutenant J. I. Johnson of the

Royal Canadian Navy have written a report of their observations which gives the best description of the condition available up to the present time. These authors suggest the following classifications of immersion foot:

1. *Minimal case:* That showing only erythema with slight sensory changes.
2. *Mild case:* That showing pitting edema, erythema, and sensory changes.
3. *Moderate case:* That showing pitting edema, erythema, blebs, and ecchymotic spots.
4. *Severe case:* That showing gross pitting edema, blebs, massive extravasations of blood, and incipient gangrene.

Treatment. Treatment may be divided into prophylaxis and treatment directed toward the correction of the condition. Prophylactic treatment consists in the removal of shoes, boots, and any constricting footwear if wet. Oil and heavy grease should be generously applied to the feet while exposed. The treatment of the condition consists in avoiding weight-bearing from the very start, avoiding any massage, and avoiding the application of heat. Absolute bed rest should be enforced; the feet should be elevated and exposed without covering, and general supporting treatment given. Locally, asepsis should be maintained and refrigeration of the extremity used. Refrigeration may be secured by the application of ice-bags or dry cooling by exposure of the feet to currents of air from an electric fan. When ice-bags are used, the skin should be protected by a covering, the entire extremity with the ice-bags wrapped in cotton, and enclosed in an oilskin bag if possible. Ice-bags should be changed every four hours, except in those cases with extreme hyperemia, in which more frequent changing will be necessary. The temperature of the feet and extremities should be maintained at around 30 to 40° F.

As a rule, within a few hours after the application of refrigeration, the patients are comfortable and edema rapidly subsides. Refrigeration should be maintained until the feet are of a healthy pink color. If blebs appear, they should be opened; if sloughs form, they must be removed. There is no advantage gained by ganglionectomy, as has been suggested, since the temperature of the feet is higher than that usually associated with sympathectomy. Most cases except those of severe grade recover completely in thirty to sixty days. The more severe type frequently results in long disability and may require amputation of toes or even the foot.

The original article, from which the above is quoted, with its colored illustrations and references, will well repay for the time spent in reading it.

March Foot

This condition, also known as march fracture, is a subperiosteal spontaneous fracture of one of the metatarsal bones, usually the second or third. This condition is completely discussed on page 269.

Summary

The conditions described are those most commonly encountered in the foot of a soldier. When these conditions occur, it should be possible by intelligent treatment to restore the men to active duty, except in the case of frost-bite, trench foot, and immersion foot, which very often reach a grade of severity which precludes any possibility of such return. Probably the greatest mistake made in military service is attempting to treat such foot conditions by halfway measures instead of by immediate hospitalization and approaching the problem from the point of view of first, relieving all acute symptoms, and second, correcting the pathology present by operation if necessary.

All of the conditions discussed except those specifically mentioned can be corrected by properly carried out conservative treatment or operation and allow return to active duty. It should be strongly emphasized, however, that it is very unwise to attempt to cure by operation a condition like bunions, spurs on the os calcis, rigid flatfoot, and rigid toe in military service, and expect a return to full active duty. The inductee with these conditions should be eliminated at once and not inducted into service unless for specified limited duty.

17

FOOT DISORDERS IN RELATION TO INDUSTRY

By reason of the large numbers engaged in industry today, the desirability, from both an economic and a humanitarian point of view, of protecting these workers from the hazards of industry and because of a real interest on the part of enlightened employers in the welfare of their employees, Industrial Medicine has become a very large and important part of medical practice. More and more physicians and nurses are seeking special training which will fit them to enter this important field and to do the job well. Certainly, there is no type of medical practice which has the opportunity of accomplishing more good and rendering greater service than is offered by Industrial Medicine, provided the training is adequate, the responsibilities involved recognized, and its obligations honestly met.

Today, practically every industrial plant employing any sizable payroll has a medical department to provide care for the employees; this as a rule is well organized, adequately staffed, and renders excellent service. Unfortunately, approximately two-thirds of the industrial workers are employed in plants with a payroll of five hundred or under; many of these plants are unable to afford their own medical departments. The biggest problem in Industrial Medicine today is that of perfecting some form of organization which will give these smaller industries an opportunity to offer their employees adequate medical care.

The primary function of the medical department in industry is to carry out pre-employment examinations, protect the workers from industrial hazards, insure healthful working conditions, maintain the general health and so the morale of the employees at as high a point as possible, and care for accidental injuries incurred during employment. In brief, its function is to reduce absenteeism due to illness or preventable causes to a minimum and to keep the employees up to the highest point of mental and physical fitness.

At the present time, there are two factors which seem likely to complicate the problem of Industrial Medicine: (1) A large number of individuals are entering industry who have never previously done manual labor, or at least have never done the type of manual labor required in industrial plants; (2) a great number of women are entering industry, doing work which may make far greater physical demands than they have ever been called upon to meet. Even after the demands of shortage of man power and economic pressure have passed, it is quite probable that women will continue to be employed in industry; consequently, the make-up of the personnel of the medical staff will probably have to be changed to meet the peculiar problems their employment will create. It is to be hoped, then, that the future will see further development in Industrial Medicine, its extension to cover small plants employing any reasonable number of individuals, and a medical personnel of sufficient diversity to cover all the major problems involved.

Functional foot disorders as a cause of lowered efficiency and even loss of employment have never, so far as the authors are aware, been studied and charted. It seems reasonable to assume, however, that the working man and woman will not differ greatly from other classes in so far as vulnerability to functional foot disorders are concerned. The prevalence of foot disorders of a degree capable of causing symptoms in college students (male) has been estimated to be 40 per cent; in women's colleges, it is probably higher. If the percentage among industrial workers is but a fraction of this, the number will be high.

From a fairly wide personal experience with this group, the impression has been gained that many industrial workers who suffer injury, particularly of the knee and lower back, have definite faults in foot attitude which commonly cause symptoms, such as undue fatigue, knee and low back pain and discomfort. Also of a large number of industrial workers claiming disability because of knee or low back pain, attributed to occupational strain, many have been relieved and their return to work made possible by the correction of obvious weight-bearing faults in the feet.

Faulty foot attitude unquestionably does cause poor posture of the feet, knees, and back; this in turn results in muscle tire because of the constant effort necessary on the part of the muscles to overcome the faulty attitude assumed. This is particularly true in occupations in which most of the day's work is performed in a limited space and in a standing position with little opportunity for moving about and changing position. Under such conditions, the same muscle groups are being constantly used and so become overworked and exhausted. When women who seldom, even while at work, care to wear a sensible shoe, are called upon to work for hours, usually at tasks which require a great deal of standing with little movement, the probability of foot strain becomes greatly increased, since the average woman's shoe lacks the supporting qualities of even the poorest shoe worn by men.

Appraisal of Foot. Pre-employment and periodic health examinations are carried out in considerable detail in well-regulated industrial medical departments. Chests and backs are x-rayed, the skin, teeth, and the nervous systems are carefully investigated, but little or nothing is said or written about the feet as a part of the investigation into the worker's physical finess. It would seem the part of wisdom, then, to include an appraisal of the capacity of the feet upon which the worker must support his weight during his working hours as part of the pre-employment or periodic health examinations which are given. This does not imply that a prospective employee should be rejected or that an employee should be denied continued employment because of faulty foot attitude. On the contrary, the finding of foot imbalance during an examination should result in helpful advice if the worker's attention is called to the condition present and the suggestion made that he consult his family physician as to what had better be done to remedy the condition for his own protection.

FOOT APPAREL IN INDUSTRY

It is a human failing to keep our best in foot, as in other apparel, for the social side of our life. Too often the worker is satisfied to wear a cheap or cast-off shoe at his work, keeping his better shoes for after hours and thereby depriving his feet of protection during those hours when they are called upon to do the most work and to sustain the greatest amount of strain. Rarely does the working man present himself for a foot examination wearing his work shoes. Nearly always it is his dress shoes that he wears, because his work shoes are not fit for public appearance. Advice as to the proper type of footwear which should be worn for the protection of the worker's feet would be helpful in almost any type of industrial plant.

There is no shoe which can be said to be a correct shoe for all types of occupations. The general principles laid down in the chapter on Foot Apparel, page 206, should be a guide for the selection of a good sensible shoe for work purposes. In addition, it may be said that a full shoe rather than an oxford should be worn, particularly by those engaged in the so-called heavy occupations, where the foot is exposed to trauma, sparks, moisture, and so forth. A heavier sole than usual is also a definite protection to the worker's feet and is therefore advisable. Shoes are manufactured which are supplied with metal caps as a protection from falling objects in certain types of occupations; such shoes afford definite protection against fractured toes and minor injuries of the foot.

A very important recent development in foot apparel for industrial workers is the manufacture of shoes with conductive soles. The purpose of such shoes is to prevent the discharge of static electrical charges through the shoes when in contact with the ground or suitably electrically conductive floors connected to the ground. The sparks resulting from such static electricity discharged in this way has led to costly and disastrous explosions. Shoes with conductive soles should be worn as a protection by workers in arsenals, flour mills, powder plants, oil plants, and many other industries in which explosive dusts or fumes are formed.

Above all, the worker should see to it that the shoes worn are in good repair and replaced often enough to insure that the foot will be protected from strain and injury. Shoes in poor repair may become industrial hazards; a loose piece of leather or a flapping shoe lace is just as readily caught in a piece of machinery as is a sleeve or other part of the clothing.

Women, as we have already stated, are a more difficult problem than are men when it comes to correct shoeing, partly because they prefer to wear what they consider a modish shoe, and partly because it is difficult to purchase on the market a common-sense shoe for women. The average woman worker's foot needs all the protection which it can be given if she is to stand up under the long hours of industry. Women workers should be instructed that high-heeled shoes, pumps, sneakers, heelless sports and rubber-soled shoes should not be worn while at work. A high-heeled shoe, particularly of the pump variety, is teetery and unstable, and is likely to lead to falls and even more serious injuries because of the insecurity of balance which results. Low or heelless shoes fail to give adequate protection to the feet for the long hours of standing and are very likely to cause undue tiring and leg and backache. Women require a higher heel than do men because their heel tendons are shorter, so that heelless or practically heelless shoes are bound to cause strain on the leg, thigh, and back muscles. A sensible oxford with a moderately high heel (page 210) will pay dividends in comfort, added efficiency, and safety.

Woolen hose are the best type of foot covering for the worker, since wool is a poor conductor of heat and readily absorbs moisture. For women, a sock interlining may be worn to protect the foot, which allows a more pleasing covering to be worn over this with comfort. Wool and silk hose should not be worn in industries which carry with them the hazard of explosion from static electricity (conductive soles), because they acquire moisture slowly and become conductors of electricity.

Needless to say, scrupulous foot hygiene is important. Daily bathing and change of hose protect the feet from uncomfortable skin eruptions, rubbing, and blistering.

Industrial workers are subject to ills of the feet other than imbalance. Rigid hammertoes, calcaneal spurs, calcaneal bursitis, bunions, tailor's bunions—in fact, all of the numerous foot abnormalities may be encountered. Such conditions can and should be remedied, for unless they are, so much unnecessary pain and discomfort will be suffered that there will be a let-down in efficiency. A word of advice from the medical department will serve to show the employee where the trouble lies and a suggestion as to its correction will often be gratefully received.

18

CONSTITUTIONAL DISEASES
AFFECTING THE FOOT

Certain constitutional conditions are important in the study of the foot because a definite part of their symptomatology is manifested in the feet. A complete discussion of these conditions would be entirely too voluminous for inclusion in a monograph of this type, but it is at least necessary briefly to discuss fundamental systemic physiologic factors which may affect the foot and departures from the normal which may occur in such physiology. The purpose of such a discussion is to point out the effects of abnormal physiologic influences on the foot and to provide a basis for making a differential diagnosis between such conditions and local functional disorders of the foot with which they may be confused, at least in the earlier stages.

If a sufficient number of patients are seen complaining of symptoms suggestive of simple foot strain, sooner or later a case will crop up, whether in private or clinic practice, in which the pathology is due, not to faulty foot architecture, but to some vascular or systemic disease. To find one's self treating a mild case of chronic vascular occlusion with a well-placed foot support is a possibility that any physician may do well to consider; the appreciation of such a pitfall will lead to a state of suspicion in examining even the most innocent-appearing case and so avoid the possibility of embarrassment at a later date.

GENERAL CONSIDERATIONS

The orthopedic surgeon is perhaps justified in considering the foot only as an organ of locomotion, but if one consults the physiologist, while not denying the above he will probably dwell instinctively on other aspects of the foot, such as its role as a medium of heat conservation or loss; as one of the four large vascular shunts, having an important place in the maintenance of blood pressure, both under normal conditions and in shock; and finally, its part as one of the interrelated units of the sympathetic nervous system. These statements one might equally well apply to the hand. However, the key factor in all of these mechanisms is the problem of circulation, and in the orthograde position of man, certain problems are posed in the position of the foot which differentiate it from the hand. These are:

1. The degree of depression of the extremity below the level of the heart; that is to say, the influence of gravity upon the circulation.
2. The extent of exposure of the foot to cold, dampness, etc.
3. The application of tight, sometimes ill-fitting accouterments to the foot.

Going further, one must appreciate that the circulatory hook-up of the foot or the hand differs primarily from that of the leg and the forearm in the following respects:

1. In the hand and foot the skin area for exposure or radiation (counting the fingers and toes) is greater in proportion to the volume of tissue contained than in the forearm or leg. It is true that the forearm and leg contain a large mass of contractile muscles, which means a greater metabolic load than is required by the soft parts in the hand and foot, and this load calls for an adequate blood supply, but the demand stays at a fairly constant level. In the hand and foot, however, because of their greater area of radiation, there is a greater variability in the demands on the circulation than is found in the forearm or leg. Functionally, then, if not actually, there is a greater flow of blood in the hands and feet than there is in the arm or leg because of this variation factor.
2. The blood vessels of the hand and foot are under the control of the vasomotor center, but the vasoconstrictor control predominates. In the forearm or leg the vasoconstrictor control is less, but there are, on the other hand, vasodilator factors to meet the demands of muscle activity. As the result of this very active and sensitive vasoconstrictor control, the blood flow in the hands and feet may be influenced to a considerable extent by hor-

monal influences and psychic and toxic stimuli; whereas, the forearm and leg will show increased blood flow only by vasodilatation or increased cardiac output.

Blood flow through the extremities depends upon the following factors:

1. Cardiac output.
2. Sympathetic control.
3. Endocrine influence.
4. Gravitational factors of position.
5. Environmental factors of heat and cold.

Cardiac Output. A discussion of cardiac output is beside the purpose of this résumé, but it should be borne in mind that with the condition of shock and fall in blood output, there follows a physiologic adjustment of vasoconstrictor impulses in the extremities, directed toward acutely reducing peripheral blood flow and directing this to vital centers. The recent work of Blalock and associates questions the value of heating the extremities in shock and thereby increasing the peripheral flow, since it is contrary to the natural impulses of conservation of cardiac output.

Sympathetic Control. The importance of the rôle of the sympathetics in peripheral circulation has been emphasized by Allen and Smithwick. Sympathetic fibers controlling the vasoconstrictor impulses in the extremity maintain circulatory pressure, shifting the flow as the need may arise, particularly in the lower extremities, since the extremities and the splanchnic area are the most sensitive areas of vasoconstriction. More important, if the flow to and from an extremity is insufficient or impaired, further afferent impulses from the adjacent vascular trunk result in reflexes which stimulate the sympathetic efferent impulses, causing further vasoconstriction and further decrease in the blood flow. One may say, then, that within limits, increased metabolic needs in any one area are met by vasoconstriction and decreased flow in another. It must be appreciated that this mechanism is set in motion by any one of a number of conditions. For example, occlusion of the popliteal artery will result in spasm of distal arterials and symptoms of claudication so that the insufficiency of the flow to the foot is actually the result of two factors: First, mechanical obstruction of the popliteal artery; and second, spasm of the distal vessels as the result of the sympathetic reflex.

The soldier standing in rigid position on a hot day, and the individual with congestive heart failure both experience diminished venous return from the lower extremities, which stimulates the sympathetics to increased vasoconstriction, for gravity makes necessary a certain amount of vasoconstriction, and poor venous return increases the necessity of extreme vasoconstriction. The entire sympathetic system is thrown into action. The excessive perspiration of the feet in hot weather does not entirely follow from nature's efforts to cool the system, but is in good part the result of sudomotor (sweat-producing) impulses, which are part and parcel of the same mechanism which produces vasoconstriction.

One may postulate varying thresholds of sympathetic release, there being lowered levels in certain individuals. Thus, the common sympathetic stimuli, such as fear or excitement, set off vasoconstriction in the extremities and vasodilatation in the face, together with sweating in the hands and in the feet. Pain may be a responsible factor, and one should appreciate the fact that a vicious cycle may be set up. The Sudeck's atrophy of the orthopedic surgeon is vasospastic dystrophy to the student of peripheral vascular disease. The pain of a sprained ankle leading to a continuous flow of afferent impulses from the diseased part brings about increasing degrees of vasospasm in the foot, gradually resulting in changes in the skin, connective tissue, muscles, and bone, so that successful treatment may require not merely healing of the initial injury, but also a break-up of the reflex sympathetic arc.

Endocrine Influence. The endocrine control of the surface flow in the foot and elsewhere lies largely within the province of thyroid physiology. The work of Stewart and Evans has shown that in patients with uncontrolled hyperthyroidism, peripheral blood flow is increased. It decreases to an appreciable degree with iodine therapy and still further with subtotal thyroidectomy. On the other hand, the myxedematous patient shows decreased blood flow, rising with elevation of the basal metabolic rate under thyroid therapy. Allen's myxedematous patients under thyroid therapy did not show any elevation of rectal temperature, indicating that the heat-control mechanism was acting peripherally. The cardiac output in myxedema is greatly lowered and is directed chiefly toward meeting the metabolic requirements of the vital organs (compare the previous note on shock), and the volume allotted to the periphery is very small. One must further consider that under such lowered rates of metabolism, heat production is greatly reduced, and this heat is conserved by decreased peripheral flow. The converse is true in hyperthyroidism. The peripheral flow and surface flow are influenced through the thyroid, acting in response to heat conservation or the necessity of increasing the heat loss.

Gravitational Factors. The influence of gravity we have mentioned. It makes necessary an element of vasoconstriction, which is counteracted to a certain extent by the active contraction of muscles, and by postural sway, both of which increase venous return. The patient suffering from the residual paralysis of poliomyelitis with an extreme degree of muscle loss presents an example of the extremity which has lost these beneficent influences. Vasoconstriction is extreme, and the clinical result is cyanosis, swelling, sweating, and claudication.

Environmental Factors. Lastly, we consider environmental factors of heat and cold. Previous chapters of this book have covered the clinical phases of exposure to cold. In this section we desire to call attention only to the influences of vasospasm and metabolic demand. Excessive exposure of the foot to cold causes vasoconstriction, as we have previously noted. If spasm reduces blood flow to the foot, the metabolic potential is lowered, and unless metabolic requirements are kept within the limits defined by the subsequent vasoconstriction, further vascular spasm and claudication will follow and may be a factor leading to gangrene. Within physiologic limits, heat increases local tissue metabolism and demands increase in peripheral blood flow. The application of heat to an extremity in which there is a reduced blood flow due to vasoconstriction is, therefore, unphysiologic and harmful.

DIAGNOSTIC METHODS

Writers on peripheral vascular disease tend to attempt definite criteria which categorically separate organic disease from functional disorders, and they have little patience with the failure of the clinician to do so. Despite their self-confidence one does well to be not only apprehensive, but humble. It does not require genius to diagnose diabetic gangrene or a badly frozen foot, but there are initial phases of the more serious organic diseases in which differentiation is far from easy. The well-organized peripheral vascular clinic tends to see referred cases at a time when signs and symptoms are more obvious.

Cramps, pains, fatigue, color disturbances, burning sensations, numbness, and tingling are considered to be classic signs of disturbed circulation. In our clinic we obtain numerous complaints of this nature in routine functional foot disorders; it must be borne in mind that a nervous 50-year-old woman in the menopause will gladly complain of all of these things after a hot day of frustrated shopping. To us the most important note is the fact that in functional disorders, the patient's feet tend to hurt only during or shortly after weight-bearing. On the other hand, leg fatigue, cramps, paresthesias, and particularly pain, carefully differentiated from generalized vague complaints or referred from other areas, may be of great significance, especially if they exist after functionally normal mechanics have been established in the foot. The simplest phases of the examination are the most informative. The foot with normal color, palpable arterial pulsation, and normal venous filling and emptying time is apt to be innocent. We are impressed with the importance of the condition of the skin and its appendages. If the nails are in reasonably good condition, and the hair of the toes and foot is normal in distribution, such evidence taken in conjunction with the above gives the clinician ample justice for proceeding at least temporarily on the basis of a local faulty foot balance. If these conditions are not met, and they should be considered in the evaluation of every foot, suspicion should be aroused and further investigation of the peripheral circulation made.

The tests of the peripheral circulation fall into four groups:

1. The oscillometer test.
2. Capillary examination.
3. Calorimetry.
4. Roentgen examination.

The oscillometer is a machine which takes a kymographic reading of the pulsation of the extremity from a cuff attached to the area in question. A somewhat similar instrument, the plethysmograph, is a more complicated device to measure the increase in blood flow in a part—a finger, for example, by placing the finger in a compartment and noting increase in the displacement of the compartment by increase in the blood flow to the parts. Both of these instruments are complicated, delicate, and expensive, and except in large specialized clinics are neither available nor particularly practical. The authors' experience with them is far from satisfactory. The oscillometer, for example, will frequently give unsatisfactory tracings of the foot and the hand, while a very beautiful tracing can be made from the calf or thigh. However, in most of the conditions in question, it is the circulation in the foot or the hand which is most important. Little is to be derived from a zero reading, and what information is obtained can readily be secured by simpler means.

Capillary microscopy, likewise, requires special equipment— in this case, a microscope with special means of illumination for examining the capillary loops in the proximal portions of the nail bed. A much simpler and yet effective means of capillary determination is that of the histamine flare test. Histamine acid phosphate 1:1000 is administered intradermally at various levels under standard conditions of temperature, noise, and exposure. Any delay in capillary response is noted.

If only one complicated, expensive instrument is to be had, the most desirable is probably a thermocouple to determine skin temperatures, since under standard conditions it reflects blood flow, and taken at various levels, the gradient of the reading will indicate the degree of loss of circulation. The element of spasm can be measured by peripheral nerve blocks followed by a second recording of the skin temperature.

Arteriography is of importance in recording the collateral circulation, the behavior of vessels in spasm, and in consequence of the above in indicating a possible level for amputation.

In addition to the above, one might finally mention the plantar ischemia test. This consists in elevating the leg to 90 degrees of flexion in recumbency. The patient then carries on active motion of the ankle, foot, and toes for one minute. The normal foot retains its color. The ischemic foot indicates occlusive vascular disease.

SYSTEMIC DISEASE SHOWING FOOT SYMPTOMS

The important clinical entities, so far as the foot is concerned, may be classified as:

1. Diseases due to vascular occlusion.
2. Diseases due to vasospasm.
3. Diseases of the hematopoietic system (bloodforming).
4. Related neurotrophic diseases.

Occlusive Vascular Disease. Occlusive vascular disease may develop as the result of either infection or degeneration. The occlusion may be generalized, or it may be the result of a clogging of a single large vessel. It may vary from acute arteritis to the development of gradual but extreme arteriosclerosis of the aged.

In the acute generalized form which follows profound general infection, the symptoms of spasm and claudication are of minor importance and rarely occur. The disease is septic in its course and is characterized by areas of purpura and hemorrhagic extravasation with subsequent development of gangrene. The old arteriosclerotic suffers from claudication, but may be completely unaware of any abnormality, even though the vessels are completely rigid as a consequence of calcareous deposit.

It is important that acute embolic vascular occlusion be recognized early, inasmuch as sympathetic block or preganglionic sympathectomy may remove a sufficient amount of the attendant spasm to prevent gangrene in the area below. Clinically, the two most important forms of occlusive vascular disease are Buerger's disease and diabetic vascular occlusion.

BUERGER'S DISEASE (THROMBO-ANGIITIS OBLITERANS). The etiology of this malady is most obscure. Buerger, who gave the most complete description of the disease, stated that it occurred almost entirely in male Jews of middle age. It is now known to occur in both sexes (predominately male), with no race distinctions, and the period of the twenties and the thirties is the age of predilection. Once the disease is present, tobacco is a factor of decided and generally recognized importance, but there is no proof that it is an etiologic factor. In this regard no positive clinical information of any importance has been developed. However, McGrath produced an experimental gangrene in rats with ergot and prevented this to a moderate degree by pre-administration of theelin. There is, however, no proof that this has any significance, clinically.

THE PATHOLOGIC FEATURES of Buerger's disease are:

1. Inflammatory reaction in the walls of the arteries.
2. Occlusive phenomena due to thrombi.
3. Canalization of the clot.
4. Low-grade inflammatory reaction, which involves other tissues locally.

The patient tends to complain of cramping pains which increase with exertion. There have been a number of clinical tests devised to induce claudication by such exertion, such as walking at a fast rate or rapid flexion and extension of the thighs on the abdomen. While pain and claudication increase with exertion, these patients do not invariably get relief from pain by rest; they may be awakened at night with cramping aches. The legs tend to be tired, cold, and subject to paresthesias.

Examination tends to show redness or cyanosis without heat, and most important of all, there is a loss of the normal moisture of the skin, inability to produce sweating, dryness of the nails, and loss of the hair over the feet and toes. Palpation may or may not reveal absence of dorsalis pedis or tibialis posticus pulse.

TREATMENT. Treatment consists in efforts to hold down metabolism in the tissues fed by the occlused circulation and to stimulate the development of collateral circulation. Locally, activity should be restricted, the foot put at rest, and kept scrupulously clean. Medical treatment consists in the use of positional exercises and intravenous therapy in the form of 2 per cent sodium citrate; this should be given slowly. In addition, the use of the Pavaex machine involving suction and pressure, and the Sanders

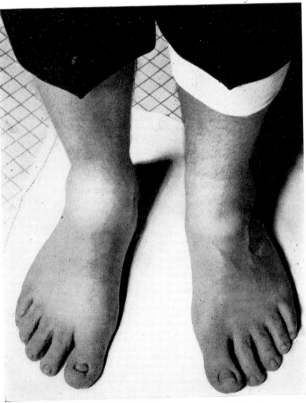

FIG. 181. Buerger's disease. Note the dark coloration of the forepart of the foot and toes.

bed to increase postural sway, are of some and often great value. Preganglionic sympathectomy is probably the most effective therapy, since it eliminates the element of vasospasm which is associated with and excited by the occlusion. By and large, the prognosis is not good. Certainly, there are very few proofs of cure, but the condition can be ameliorated and kept to a minimum by intelligent management. It may be reasonably said that fewer amputations are performed today than previously due to improved methods of treatment, chiefly in the direction of surgery on the sympathetic system.

DIABETES. Any patient with any degree of circulatory impairment, particularly of the extremities, should be suspected of diabetes—at least to the extent of having several urine determinations carried out. A urine, positive for sugar, should lead to further examinations of blood sugar and fractionation studies on 24-hour urine specimens. The symptoms in the beginning are tingling and numbness in the feet with discoloration of one or more toes, and, at times, progressive gangrene may occur due to interference with the circulation.

TREATMENT. Naturally, a positive finding of sugar in the urine and increased blood sugar should lead to an effort to control the metabolic disease, since control of a diabetes itself has a profound effect upon the future of the peripheral vascular disease. Local measures do not differ greatly from those mentioned in connection with the treatment of Buerger's disease. Gangrenous toes, an entire foot, or even the leg may require amputation.

LUETIC ENDO-ARTERITIS. Luetic endo-arteritis should be borne in mind. One case has been seen with symptoms fairly typical of a Buerger's disease in which a complete arrest and normal restoration of function followed the use of the Pavaex and specific treatment. This patient has been free of all symptoms for over one year.

Vasospastic Disturbances. These conditions are the result of vasomotor instability. In this group may be found cases with mild vasomotor instability and more severe types, such as Raynaud's disease, acrocyanosis, and erythromelalgia. These severe forms are rare in the utmost degree.

RAYNAUD'S DISEASE. The symptoms and complications of Raynaud's disease arise as the result of an exaggerated sympathetic response to a normal stimulus. This stimulus may be emotional excitement, exposure to cold, sexual or mental disorders, trauma, etc. In its classic form, Raynaud's disease is characterized by a series of events termed the "color cycle." This cycle consists of repeated attacks of symmetrical involvement of the arms and legs, particularly the upper extremities (the latter in females), in which the extremity first becomes blanched or wax-like, followed by a cycle of cyanosis, and finally by a cycle of redness. Capillary microscopy has indicated that the first stage is due to spasm of the arterials. The loops are incompletely filled, and the capillaries have a broken appearance, due to the passing through of few corpuscles. The collecting venules are not well visualized. The second stage consists in a back flow from the more or less relaxed venules. The capillaries at this stage are more numerous, and there appears to be some stagnation in the capillary loops as the result of blood entering from both the arterial and the venous sides. The third stage of redness consists in a mild inflammatory reaction to the previous condition. The period of redness is associated with a burning pain. In extreme cases, local gangrene of the tips of the toes occurs, and intractable ulcers develop.

TREATMENT. Mild cases may be controlled by the management of any causative factor which can be determined, usually a nervous instability. The more severe cases require pre-ganglionic sympathectomy. The importance of the sympathetics in this disease has been well brought out by Smithwick, who has reported a patient, a skier, who under normal conditions experienced attacks on exposure to cold. After sympathectomy, the girl found that after a short time in the cold atmosphere, the affected hand was colder than the normal hand, but after prolonged exposure to cold, the affected hand felt warm and comfortable, while the normal hand became cold and cramped.

ACROCYANOSIS. There is little occasion to describe or use the term "acrocyanosis" as a special clinical entity, since acrocyanosis arises under the same circumstances and is to be differentiated from Raynaud's disease only by the fact that the color cycle does not occur, and the fact that it is of milder degree. One observer has emphasized the fact that in acrocyanosis there is elevation of venous pressure, which is not found in Raynaud's syndrome. This, however, has not been confirmed.

ERYTHROCYANOSIS. Erythrocyanosis has been described by Lewis as a reddish, cyanotic appearance of the skin of the legs, attributed to extensive reaction to cold. It is likely that this also is part of the same mechanism as found in the previous disorders, the local vascular reaction being one of capillary dilation. It is to be noted that there is no heat present, and that it is likely that sympathetic reaction causes vasoconstriction of the deeper structures while the capillaries are dilated. The application of heat increases the pain and vasoconstriction. The problem presented by this condition in no way differs from that of the more common forms of vasospasm following exposure to cold.

The Hematopoietic System. (Blood forming.) Two blood dyscrasias are likely to result in changes in the foot. These are polycythemia vara and hemorrhagic purpura.

POLYCYTHEMIA VARA. This condition results in increased blood volume, the effect being greater on the large veins, in both the viscera and the extremities. There is pain in the foot, the temperature of the skin is not increased, but the active saturation of the venous and arterial blood is increased. A blood count will usually reveal the obvious nature of the condition.

HEMORRHAGIC PURPURA. In purpura fulminans, there is a clinical picture of acute infection with early appearance of ecchymosis and hemorrhagic extravasations. The upper extremities as well as the lower extremities are involved, and the body also. This is a disease of children, and it is questionable whether it is actually of purpura hemorrhagica or some overwhelming form of arterial infection.

Diseases of the Nervous System. Certain diseases of the nervous system are associated with foot symptoms. The symptoms are chiefly those of mild numbness, tingling, and paresthesia in the feet. Pernicious anemia is the chief disease of the nervous system which gives rise to foot symptoms.

PERNICIOUS ANEMIA. In pernicious anemia the numbness, tingling, and paresthesia tend to be symmetrical, sometimes associated with loss of muscle control. There is also some evidence of nutritional deficiency. There is evidence of disturbance of the position sense and an impaired sense of vibration. The picture may vary all the way from that of spastic paralysis through that of posterolateral sclerosis. These disturbances in the feet are not the result of hematopoietic disorder in itself, but are the result of degeneration in the myelin sheaths of the posterior columns of the cord and axis cylinders.

TREATMENT. Recent investigations have indicated that vitamin B_1—that is, thiamine—is of great importance in these conditions, since they are likely to be present not only in pernicious anemia, but also in chronic alcoholism, gastric carcinoma, obstructions and fistulae of the intestinal tracts, scurvy, pellagra, and hemorrhagic icterus. In all of these conditions there is a loss of gastric acidity and nutritional deficiency. It has recently been shown that thiamine has a beneficial effect on the residual manifestations of primary pernicious anemia over and above the effect of liver. It is felt that thiamine is of importance as a catalyst in the intermediary metabolism of carbohydrates, particularly in the nerve sheaths, and that the nerve degeneration results from disturbance of the CHO metabolism.

19

FOOT STRAPPING

While strapping with adhesive tape is a very efficient method of giving support to a painful foot, it should be used only as a temporary measure. Prolonged strapping tends to weaken the supporting structures of the foot and may cause uncomfortable and even dangerous irritation.

The preliminary preparation for strapping the foot or ankle should be carefully made to avoid irritation and unnecessary discomfort. The foot and ankle should be carefully shaved and thoroughly cleansed with benzine or ether.

BASKET STRAPPING

This type of strapping is the most universally used. It is recommended for sprains of the ankle, sprains of the subastragaloid joint, and sprains of the tarsus. It is also useful for an acutely painful foot due to foot strain or mild inflammatory infection in the joints of the tarsus.

A strip of adhesive one inch wide is used. The patient is seated with the knee slightly flexed and the foot is held at a right angle to the leg and slightly adducted (Fig. 182A). This position of the foot is maintained by passing a bandage under the ball of the foot and having the patient hold the ends. The first strip of adhesive starts from a point four to six inches above the external malleolus well posterior and passes under the posterior part of the heel and up the inner side of the leg four to six inches above the internal malleolus (Fig. 182B). The second strip is carried from the base of the fifth toe, along the lateral side of the foot and around the heel to the base of the great toe on the medial side of the foot (Fig. 182C). The third strip starts at a point slightly anterior to the first strip, follows its general line, slightly overlapping it. The fourth strip begins at a point one-half to one inch behind and above the second strip, following its direction and slightly overlapping to terminate about one-half inch behind this strip, on the inner side of the foot. Successive strips are applied in this manner until the vertical strips reach a point about one inch in front of the internal and external malleoli and the horizontal strips reach a point one inch above the mal-

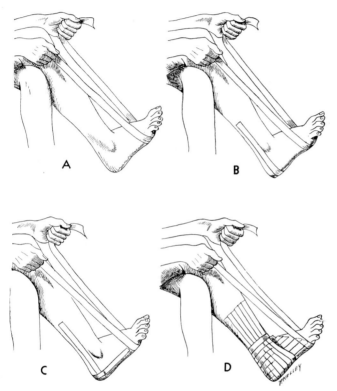

FIG. 182. Basket strapping of the foot and ankle. A, position of foot for strapping; B-C, method of applying the vertical and longitudinal strips; D, strapping completed.

leoli. The strapping should never completely encircle the ankle or foot at any point. The entire strapping should be covered with a two-inch roller bandage for several hours to prevent slipping of the adhesive, after which it may be removed. The strapping should be replaced or tightened every three or four days until the acute symptoms subside.

LONGITUDINAL ARCH STRAPPING

(Fig. 183.) This type of strapping may be used for pronation of the foot when acute pain is complained of in the longitudinal arch. The foot is held dorsiflexed at a right angle to the leg and slightly adducted. One-inch adhesive is used. The first strip of adhesive starts at a point behind the external malleolus and is

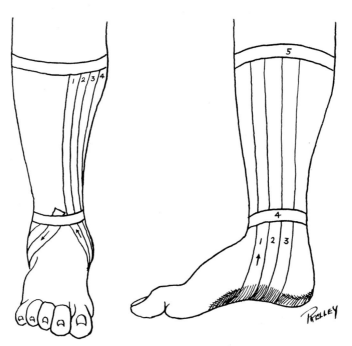

FIG. 183. Longitudinal arch strapping, used in acute foot strain.

carried around the heel and up the medial side of the leg to a point about six or seven inches above the internal malleolus and slightly behind it. The second strip begins on the outer side of the leg at a point anterior to and slightly overlapping the first and ending on the medial side of the leg anteriorly and slightly overlapping. Two or three more strips are applied in this manner until they reach a point slightly anterior to the malleoli. A circular strapping is applied two inches above the malleoli and at the terminal of the strapping on the medial side of the leg. This strapping should be covered with a two-inch roller bandage to hold the adhesive in place. This strapping tends to overcome the pronated position of the foot and to shift the body weight toward the lateral side of the foot. The strapping should be replaced or tightened every three or four days until the acute pain subsides.

MORTON STRAPPING

Dr. D. J. Morton has described a unique method of strapping which may be used for sprains of the ankle, subastragaloid, and tarsal joints. This type of strapping may also be used in cases of flat or weak feet when acute pain is complained of. The strapping, if properly applied, will tend to overcome pronation and elevate the longitudinal arch.

Strips of adhesive one inch wide are used (Fig. 184). The knee on the affected side is flexed, and the foot is held dorsiflexed to a right angle and slightly adducted. The first strip starts two inches above the internal malleolus (Fig. 184[1]), and is carried down across the sole of the foot, crossing the base of the fifth metatarsal. It is then carried over the dorsum of the foot (Fig. 184[2]), crossing the instep over the scaphoid bone, around the heel slightly below the internal malleolus, and along the upper border of the os calcis. The strip then passes obliquely around the lateral side of the heel and sole, tension being made to adduct the heel slightly. The strip is then carried under the heel and up the medial side of the ankle anterior to it but overlapping its beginning (Fig. 184[3]). The second strip begins at a point over the external malleolus, overlapping the first strip, and passes over the dorsum and around the heel. It is then carried obliquely forward (Fig. 184[4-5]), around and under the heel and up on the medial side of the foot, ending with one and one-quarter circular turns (Fig. 184[6]) on a level just above the malleoli. The third strip is applied to the second which it overlaps by half its width posteriorly as far as the dorsum, then overlies it until approaching the circular turns, which overlap half width above the previous one (Fig. 184[7-8]). The foot is freely movable in all directions except pronation. If the strapping

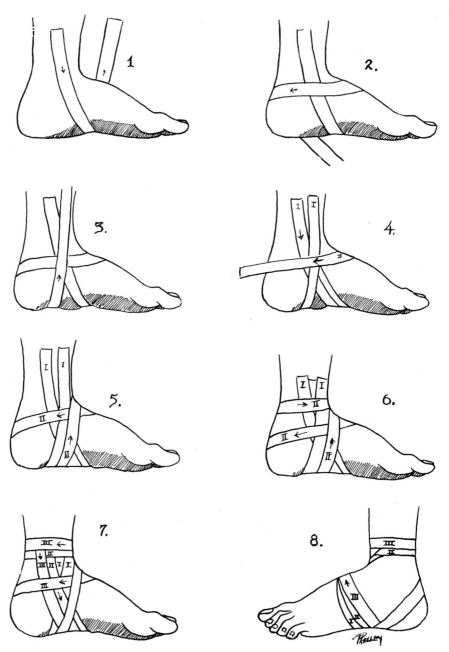

Fɪɢ. 184. Morton's strapping. (See text for complete description of application.)

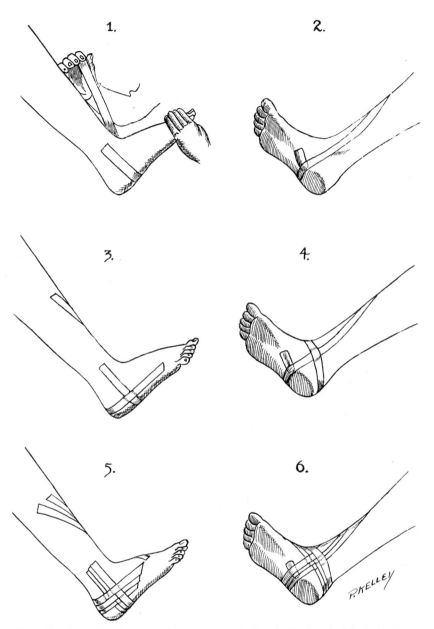

FIG. 185. Strapping for acute foot strain in the longitudinal arch. Method of application.

is properly applied, there is little danger of interfering with circulation. Do not apply the circular bands too tightly.

STRAPPING FOR ACUTE FOOT STRAIN

This standardized army method of strapping, slightly modified by Frieberg and Jones, is used chiefly in acute foot strain when pain is complained of in the longitudinal arch of the foot (Fig. 185). The foot is held in a dorsiflexed position with the sole slightly inverted. (1) A small piece of soft wool felt some two inches by three inches is held just below the head of the astragalus and the scaphoid. (2) Strips of one-inch adhesive tape are used. The first strip is attached just above the external malleolus, passes under the heel, and up over the felt pad and astragalus, ending over the shin (Fig. 185[1-2]). The second strip is attached over the head of the fifth metatarsal, passes parallel with the sole of the foot and around the heel and forward to the dorsal aspect of the foot, which anchors the foot in adduction. Successive layers of adhesive strips are superimposed upon these two, overlapping them about one-fourth of their width. The upper ends of the long strips that go up the shin spread out fan-shaped to give greater area of skin attachment and better support.

METATARSAL ARCH STRAPPING

This method of strapping is used in acute anterior metatarsalgia when the pain is localized between or at the base of the toes (Fig. 186). The foot is held dorsiflexed at a right angle with the toes forcibly flexed (Fig. 186[1]). Three or four one-inch adhesive strips are used. The first strip is carried around the ball of the foot with its forward margin falling just behind the heads of the first and fifth metatarsal bones. The second and third strips are applied in the same circular manner, slightly overlapping the previously applied strip. The strips should not completely encircle the foot but one-half inch space should be left between the ends (Fig. 186[2-3]). A small metatarsal pad of soft wool felt may be placed just posterior to the metatarsal heads (Fig. 186[4]). This strapping, if properly applied, will tend to hold the meta-

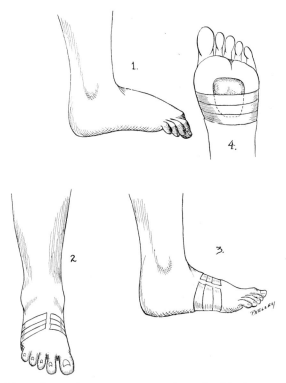

Fig. 186. Type of strapping to support anterior arch of foot: 1, position of foot and toes for strapping; 2 and 3, views of strapping; 4, soft felt anterior heel can be incorporated in strapping for support.

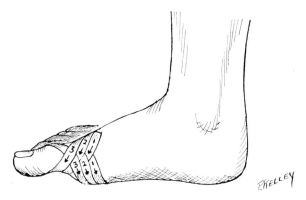

Fig. 187. Spica strapping of the great toe. Used in injury and inflammation of the great toe joint.

tarsal heads in their normally arched position and relieve the acute pain which accompanies a depressed anterior arch.

SPICA STRAPPING OF THE GREAT TOE

In cases of acute pain in the great toe joint such as is experienced in hallux rigidus, arthritis, and injury, a spica strapping applied around the great toe joint will partially immobilize the joint and tend to relieve the pain (Fig. 187). One-half inch strips are used; the first strip encircles the great toe joint in a spiral direction on its medial side; the second encircles the lateral side of the toe in the same manner. Successive strips are applied, slightly over-lapping.

20

FOOT EXERCISES

The efficient functioning of the foot is dependent upon both structural and postural stability. Structural stability is dependent upon a normal foot architecture and normal supporting ligaments. Postural stability is dependent upon the leg being maintained in a functionally vertical plane over the foot so that the superimposed weight may be distributed equally over the foot with the body at rest and in motion. Muscle balance or equality in the strength of antagonistic muscles or muscle groups is essential to the maintenance of postural stability, since both the long muscles passing across the ankle joint and the intrinsic muscles of the foot are the agencies which maintain the leg in a balanced position over the foot. Functional foot disorders, the result of faulty foot attitudes, throw an abnormal strain upon these muscles which become eventually weakened and unable to function efficiently. By the use of supports and balanced shoes, faulty foot attitudes may be corrected, and the supporting muscles relieved of strain; and they can be restored to their normal tone and power by systematic building up exercises.

The following exercises have proved effective in stretching contracted muscles and improving the power in those weakened by disuse or overuse.

The exercises which follow should be carried out twice daily, preferably morning and evening, and of course always in the bare feet.

EXERCISE NO. 1

FLEXION AND EXTENSION EXERCISES

This exercise develops the musculature which supports the long arch of the foot.

Position: Sitting with legs crossed.

Action: Fully extend (Fig. 188), then fully flex the foot at the ankle, turning the sole of the foot in as far as possible (Fig. 189), and keep the toes extended in both positions.

Repeat the exercise ten to twenty times.

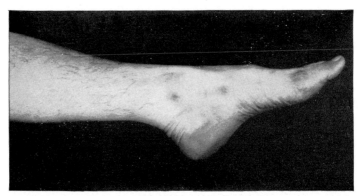

Fig. 188

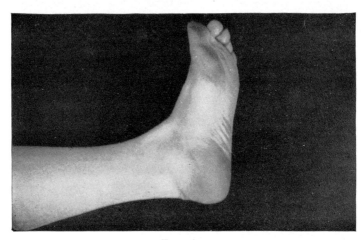

Fig. 189

EXERCISE NO. 2

TOE SPREADING EXERCISE

This exercise develops the muscles which support the anterior or metatarsal arch of the foot.

POSITION: Sitting, resting the heel on the floor.

ACTION: Forcibly flex the toes and invert the foot slightly (Fig. 190). Hold the foot in this position for a few seconds, then extend and spread the toes as far as possible (Fig. 191). Hold this position for a few seconds, then complete the exercise by flexing the toes into the original position.

Repeat the exercise ten to twenty times.

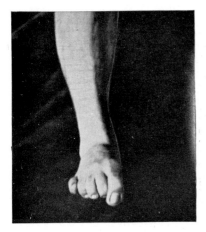 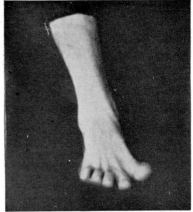

FIG. 190   FIG. 191

EXERCISE NO. 3

TOE GRIPPING EXERCISE

This exercise develops the musculature which supports the metatarsal arch of the foot.

POSITION: Sitting with several marbles or jackstones on the floor.

ACTION: Grasp the marble or jackstone with the toes and pick it up, placing it a foot or so from its original position. Now replace the marbles to their original position with the other foot. (Figs. 192, 193.)

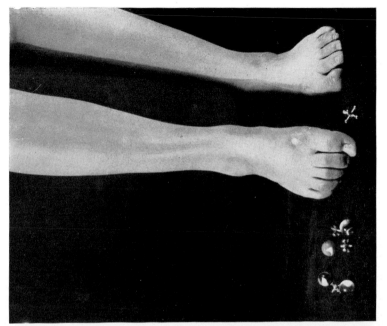

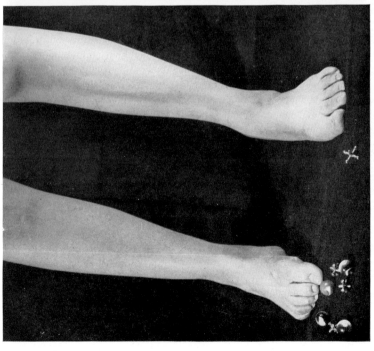

EXERCISE NO. 4

FOOT ADDUCTION EXERCISE (Standing)

This exercise develops the adductor muscles of the feet which aid in maintaining proper balance of the longitudinal arch.

POSITION: Standing with hands on hips, feet parallel and about four inches apart (Fig. 194).

ACTION: Keeping the toes and heels firmly on the floor, slightly bend the knees and gradually separate them by rolling the knees outward (Fig. 195). Return to the original position, and repeat ten times.

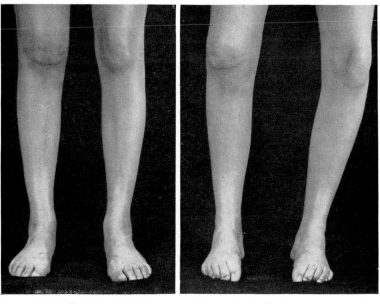

FIG. 194   FIG. 195

EXERCISE NO. 5

FOOT ADDUCTION EXERCISE (Walking)

This exercise stretches the muscles on the lateral side of the foot and strengthens the muscles on the medial side of the foot, which tends to hold the arches in the proper position. This is an excellent exercise to overcome weak feet.

POSITION: Standing, ready to take a step. The foot is rolled to the outer side and the toes forcibly flexed. (Figs. 196, 197.)

ACTION: Take twenty-five to fifty steps with the foot in this position.

This position holds both the longitudinal and the metatarsal arches in their exaggerated proper positions.

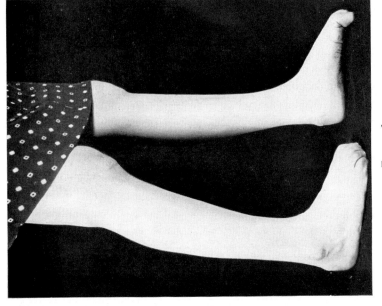

FIG. 197

FIG. 196

EXERCISE NO. 6

HEEL STRETCHING EXERCISE (Sitting)

This exercise stretches the heel tendons which in most cases of weak feet are short and strengthens the muscle groups which hold the long arch in place.

POSITION: Sitting with the foot flat on the floor (Fig. 198).

ACTION: Flex the foot upward on the ankle, flexing the toes downward and pulling the foot inward. Pull the foot up and in as far as possible (Fig. 199). Now complete the exercise by slowly lowering the foot to its original position.

The exercise should be performed ten to twenty times with each foot. Keep the heel stationary on the floor.

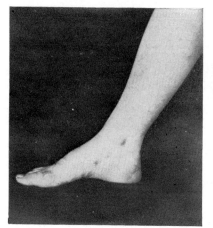
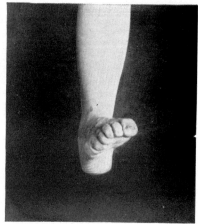

FIG. 198   FIG. 199

EXERCISE NO. 7

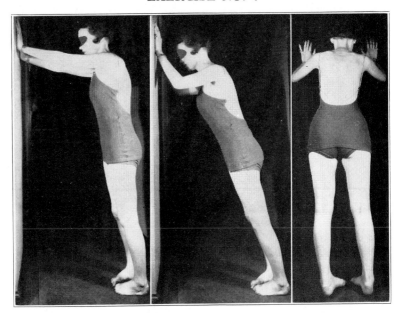

FIG. 200   FIG. 201   FIG. 202

HEEL STRETCHING EXERCISE (Standing)

This exercise stretches the heel tendon and strengthens the muscle groups which hold the arches in balance.

POSITION: Standing, facing, and three or four feet from the wall. Toes are turned in and forcibly flexed, and the body weight is rolled to the outer side of the foot (Fig. 200).

ACTION: Lean on the wall with arms straight, back rigid, and head erect. Slowly flex the arms, keep the back straight, and knees and hips extended and heels firmly on the floor until the head touches the wall, or as nearly as is possible, rolling the feet to the outer side (Figs. 201, 202). Hold this position for a few seconds, then slowly straighten the arms, assuming the original position. Repeat this movement ten to twenty times.

If the exercise is properly done the patient feels a distinct pulling in the calf and thigh of the leg.

BIBLIOGRAPHY

TEXTBOOKS CONSULTED

Albee, F. H.: Orthopedic Surgery, Philadelphia, W. B. Saunders Co., 1919.

Bradford, E. H. and R. W. Lovett: Orthopedic Surgery, Baltimore, William Wood, 1915.

Campbell, W. C.: A Text Book on Orthopedic Surgery, Philadelphia, W. B. Saunders Co., 1930.

Cunningham, D. J.: Text Book of Anatomy, Baltimore, William Wood, 1913.

Davis, G. G.: Applied Anatomy, Philadelphia, J. B. Lippincott Co., 1924.

Dickson, F. D.: Posture, Philadelphia, J. B. Lippincott Co., 1931.

Gray, H.: Anatomy, Philadelphia, Lea and Febiger, 1936.

Jamieson, E. B.: Regional Anatomy, Baltimore, William Wood, 1936.

Jones, Sir R. L. and R. W. Lovett: Orthopedic Surgery, Baltimore, William Wood, 1929.

Lake, N. C.: The Foot, Baltimore, William Wood, 1935.

Lewin, P.: Orthopedic Surgery for Nurses, Philadelphia, W. B. Saunders Co., 1928.

Mercer, W.: Orthopedic Surgery, Baltimore, William Wood, 1933.

Morton, D. J.: The Human Foot, New York, Columbia University Press, 1935.

Nutt, J. J.: Diseases and Deformities of the Foot, New York, E. B. Treat Co., 1925.

Shands, A. R.: Handbook of Orthopedic Surgery, St. Louis, C. V. Mosby, 1937.

Steindler, A.: Operative Orthopedics, New York, D. Appleton Co., 1925.

Sutton, R. L. and R. L. Sutton, Jr.: Diseases of the Skin, St. Louis, C. V. Mosby Co., 1935.

Walter, H. E.: The Human Skeleton, New York, Macmillan Co., 1918.

Whitman, R.: Orthopedic Surgery, 2d ed., 1903; 3d ed., 1907; 7th ed., 1923; 8th ed., Philadelphia, Lea and Febiger, 1927.

ACCESSORY SCAPHOID

Kidner, F. C.: Jour. Bone and Joint Surg., 11:831, 1929.

AFFECTIONS OF THE HEEL

Allison, N.: Jour. Bone and Joint Surg., 6:91, 1924.

Chang, C. C. and Miltner, L. J.: Jour. Bone and Joint Surg., 16:355, 1934.

Hertzler, A. E.: Amer. Jour. Surg., 1:117, 1926.

Lewin, P.: Surg., Gynec. and Obst., 41:579, 1925.

Lewin, P.: Arch. Surg., 12:117, 1926.

Meyerding, T. W. and Stuck, W. G.: Jour. Amer. Med. Asso., 102:1658, 1834.

Roberts, P. W.: Jour. Bone and Joint Surg., 11:338, 1929.

Sever, J. W.: N. Y. Med. Jour., 95:1025, 1912.

ATHLETE'S FOOT

Gilman, R. L.: Jour. Amer. Med. Asso., 100:715, 1933.

Muskatblit, E.: N. Y. State Med. Jour., 33:632, 1933.

White, R. P.: Brit. Jour. Dermatol., 44:489, 1932.

CORNS

Chase, H. M.: Boston Med. and Surg. Jour., 175:134, 1916.

Galland, W. I.: Jour. Amer. Med. Asso., 100:880, 1933.

EVOLUTIONARY DEVELOPMENT OF THE FOOT

Engle, E. T. and D. J. Morton: Jour. Bone and Joint Surg., 13:311, 1931.
Keith, A.: Jour. Bone and Joint Surg., 11:10, 1929.

EXERCISES

Bettmann, E.: Jour. Bone and Joint Surg., 19:821, 1937.
Dickson, F. D., and R. L. Diveley: Exercises for Health and Correction, Philadelphia, J. B. Lippincott Co., 1923.

FLATFOOT

White, J. Warren: Jour. Bone and Joint Surg., 22:547-554, 1940.
Young, Charles S.: Surg., Gynec., and Obstet., 68:1099-1101, 1939.

FOOT OF ADOLESCENT

Butte, F. L.: Jour. Bone and Joint Surg., 19:496, 1937.
Hoke, M.: Jour. Bone and Joint Surg., 13:773, 1931.
Miller, O. L.: Jour. Bone and Joint Surg., 9:84, 1927.
Steindler, A.: Jour. Orth. Surg., 2:8, 1920.

FOOT APPAREL

Adams, J. D.: Jour. Amer. Med. Asso., 92:1753, 1929.
Buka, A. J.: Jour. Amer. Med. Asso., 93:445, 1929.
Cranor, K. T.: Hygeia, 9:937, 1931.
Munson, E. L.: The Soldier's Foot and the Military Shoe, Ft. Leavenworth, Kans. 1912.
Painter, C. F.: Boston Med. and Surg. Jour., 197:254, 1927.
Schwartz, R. P.: Physiother. Rev., 13:105, 1933.

FOOT OF CHILDHOOD

Brahdy, M. B.: Arch. Pediatr., 44:86, 1927.
Elmslie, R. C.: The Practitioner, 125:195, 1930.
Lewin, P.: Amer. Jour. Dis. Child., 31:704, 1926.
Reading, H. E.: Intern. Clin., 4:139, 1930.
Roberts, P. W.: Jour. Amer. Med. Asso., 75:237, 1920.
Roehm, H. R.: Arch. Pediatr., 50:380, 1933.
Schneider, C. C.: Wis. Med. Jour., 25:284, 1926.
Schumm, H. C.: Amer. Jour. Dis. Child., 38:1273, 1929.

FOOT IMBALANCE

Abbott, E. G. and Pingree, H. A.: N. Y. Med. Jour., 87:875, 1908.
Ashley, D. D.: Med. Rec., 140:654, 1934.
Berg, R. F.: West. Jour. Surg., 39:261, 1931.
Betts, L. O.: Med. Jour. Australia, 1:1940.
Brockman, E. P.: The Clinical Jour., 57:109, 1928.
Caldwell, G. A.: Hygeia, 8:631, 1930.
Conn, H. R.: Jour. Ind. Hyg., 9:77, 1927.
Corbusier, H. D.: Amer. Med., 23:328, 1917.
Dodd, H.: Brit. Jour. Surg., 21:131, 1933.
Dunn, H. L.: Amer. Jour. Hyg., 8:410, 1928.

Fischer, E.: Jour. Bone and Joint Surg., 19:185, 1937.
Forbes, A. M.: Amer. Jour. Orth. Surg., 8:507, 1911.
Forrester-Brown, M.: Brit. Med. Jour., 1:463, 1932.
Geist, E. S.: Surg. Clin. N. Amer., 3:1389, 1923.
Gottlieb, A.: Amer. Jour. Phys. Ther., 8:41, 1931.
Haggart, G. E.: Surg. Clin. N. Amer., 11:371, 1931.
Harris, J. R.: Milit. Surgeon, 34:1, 1914.
Hatch, E. S.: New Orleans Med. and Surg. Jour., 75:294, 1922.
Humphries, R. E. and Taylor, G. H.: Amer. Jour. Surg., 7:808, 1929.
Hyman, E.: New Orleans Med. and Surg. Jour., 84:861, 1932.
Kurtz, A. D.: Jour. Med. Soc. New Jersey, 29:686, 1932.
Kyle, B. H.: Jour. Bone and Joint Surg., 7:722, 1925.
Lewin, P.: Jour. Amer. Med. Asso., 88:994, 1927.
Lord, J. P.: Jour. Amer. Med. Asso., 81:1502, 1923.
Mebane, T. S.: Milit. Surgeon, 47:428, 1920.
Mitchell, T. J.: Med. Rec., 81:896, 1912.
Morton, D. J.: Jour. Bone and Joint Surg., 6:368, 1924.
Morton, D. J.: Jour. Bone and Joint Surg., 19:1052, 1937.
Oxford, T. M.: Painful Feet, New Orleans Med. and Surg. Jour., 89:86-92, 1936.
Peabody, C. W.: Physiother. Rev., 12:79, 1932.
Rechtman, A. M.: Hygeia, 7:479, 1929.
Reed, E. N.: Jour. Bone and Joint Surg., 16:471, 1934.
Smith, E.: N. Y. Med. Jour., 109:225, 1919.
Wheeler, H. L.: Milit. Surg., 78:438, 1936.
Whitman, A.: N. Y. St. Jour. Med., 30:319, 1930.
Whitman, R.: Amer. Jour. Orth. Surg., 11:215, 1913
Wiles, P.: Brit. Med. Jour., 2:563, 1933.
Winsor, H.: Amer. Med., 37:364, 1931.

FOOT STRAPPING

Morton, D. J.: Milit. Surgeon, 42:450, 1918.

HALLUX VALGUS

Bradford, E. H.: Amer. Jour. Orth. Surg., 12:169, 1914.
Galland, W. I.: Surg., Gynec. and Obst., 66:95, 1938.
Girdlestone, G. R. and Spooner, H. J.: Jour. Bone and Joint Surg., 19:30, 1937.
Jones, Robt.: Brit. Med. Jour., 2:651, 1924.
Keller, W. L.: N. Y. Med. Jour., 80:741, 1904.
Keller, W. L.: N. Y. Med. Jour., 95:696, 1912.
Kleinberg, S.: Amer. Jour. Surg., 15:75, 1932.
Lapidus, P. W.: Surg. Gynec. and Obst., 58:183, 1934.
Mayo, C. H.: Ann. Surg., 48:300, 1908.
McBride, E. D.: Jour. Bone and Joint Surg., 10:735, 1928.
McBride, E. D.: Jour. Amer. Med. Asso., 105:1164, 1935.
McMurray, T. P.: Brit. Med. Jour., 2:218, 1936.
Peabody, C. W.: Jour. Bone and Joint Surg., 13:273, 1931.
Roberts, P. W.: Jour. Amer. Med. Asso., 80:540, 1923.
Silver, D.: Jour. Bone and Joint Surg., 5:225, 1923.
Singley, J. D.: Jour. Amer. Med. Asso., 61:1871, 1913.
Stanley, L. L. and Breck, L. W.: Jour. Bone and Joint Surg., 17:961, 1935.
Truslow, W.: Jour. Bone and Joint Surg., 7:98, 1925.

HALLUX VARUS

Haas, S. L.: Jour. Bone and Joint Surg., **20**:705-708, 1938.

HAMMERTOE

Young, Charles S.: Jour. Bone and Joint Surg., **20**: 1938.

IMMERSION FOOT

Webster, D. R., F. M. Woolhouse, and J. L. Johnston: Jour. Bone and Joint Surg., **24**:785-794, 1942.

INFRACTION OF THE SECOND METATARSAL BONE

Frieberg, A. H.: Jour. Bone and Joint Surg., **8**:257, 1926.
Mouchet, A.: Jour. Bone and Joint Surg., **11**:87, 1929.
Painter, C. F.: Boston Med. and Surg. Jour., **184**:533, 1921.

INGROWN TOE NAILS

Graham, H. F.: Amer. Jour. Surg., **6**:411, 1929.
Keyes, E. L.: Jour. Amer. Med. Asso., **102**:1458, 1934.
Winograd, A. M.: Jour. Amer. Med. Asso., **92**:229, 1929.

KOHLER'S DISEASE

Karp, M. G.: Jour. Bone and Joint Surg., **19**:84, 1937.
Kidner, F. C. and Muro, F.: Jour. Amer. Med. Asso., **83**:1650, 1924.
Köhler, A.: Arch. Klin. Chir., **101**:560, 1913.
Köhler, A.: Tenth. Rontg. Kong., Fort. Gebiete Rontstr., in Münch Med. Wchnschr., **67**:1289, 1920.
Köhler, A.: Amer. Jour. Roentgenol., **10**:705, 1923.

MARCH FOOT

Blauvelt, H.: Brit. Med. Jour., **1**:1218, 1935.
Breithaupt: Med. Zeitg., **24**:169, 1855.
Dodd, H.: Brit. Jour. Surg., **21**:131, 1933.
Elward, J. F.: Amer. Jour. Roentgenol., **36**:188, 1936.
Goldman, S. E.: Jour. Bone and Joint Surg., **10**:228, 1928.
Jansen, M.: Jour. Bone and Joint Surg., **8**:262, 1926.
Maseritz, I. H.: Arch. Surg., **32**:49, 1936.
Sloane, D. and Sloane, M. F.: Amer. Jour. Surg., **31**:167, 1936.
Speed, J. S. and H. B. Macey: Jour. Bone and Joint Surg., **15**:903, 1933.
Straus, F. H.: Surg., Gynec. and Obst., **54**:581, 1932.

PHYSIOLOGY

Schwartz, R. P., et al.: Jour. Bone and Joint Surg., **16**:343, 1934; **19**:431, 1937.

SESAMOID BONES

Hobart, M. H.: Jour. Bone and Joint Surg., **2**:298, 1929.
Inge, G. A. and Ferguson, A. B.: Arch. Surg., **27**:466, 1933.

INDEX

Page numbers in **bold face** type indicate pages on which
pertinent illustrations appear

Bunion—(*Continued*)
    treatment of—(*Continued*)
        operative—(*Continued*)
            Mayo operation, 228
            McBride operation, 233
        prophylactic, 222
        x-ray picture of, **217**
Bunion protectors, 223
Bursa, of heel, **284**
    operation for removal of, **225**
    retrocalcaneal, inflammation of, 283
Bursitis, 283, 295
    treatment of, 283

Calcaneal spurs, see Heel, affections of
Calcaneobursitis, **284**
Calcium, deficiency of, as factor in
        imbalance, 102
    treatment for, 102
Callosities, as evidence of imbalance,
        112, 113
    in flatfoot, 159
    in high-arched foot, 185
    in mallet toe, 245
Callus, 258
    definition of, 258
Chilblains, 296
Chimpanzee, foot of, compared with
        human foot, **7**
Civilization as contributing cause of
        foot strain, 147
Clavus, see Callus and Corns
Club nail, 255, **256**
    etiology of, 255
    treatment of, 255
        removal of, 257
Cod-liver oil, in treatment of calcium
        deficiency, 102
Constitutional diseases affecting feet,
        see Foot, diseases of, constitutional
Corns, 258, **259**
    definition of, 258
    etiology of, 259
    as evidence of imbalance, 112, 113
    soft, 261
        treatment of, 261
    symptoms of, 259
    treatment of, conservative, 260
        operative, 260
Cramps, in calves of legs due to muscle
        strain, 157
Cuboid bones, anatomy of, 12

Cuneiform bones, anatomy of, 12
    evolutionary development of, 5

Diabetes, 316
Diet, in treatment of imbalance, 102
Dorsalis pedis artery, 31

Eczema, 266
    treatment of, 266
Endocrine glands, disturbances of, as
        etiologic factors in imbalance, 101
Epiphysitis, of os calcis, see Heel, affec-
        tions of, calcaneal apophysitis
Equilibrium, sense of, in children be-
        ginning to walk, 68
    significance in posture, 34
Equinocavus position of foot in high-
        arched foot, 184
Erythromelalgia, 317
Examination, general physical, indica-
        tions for, 58
    family history, 57
    history of present illness, 57
Examination of foot, examining stand,
        59
    gait, 63
    general, 60
    heel tendon, 62
    imbalance in childhood, 90
    longitudinal arch, 61
    metatarsal arch, 61
    pedograph, 63
    plantar fascia, 63
    position of examiner and patient, **60**
    relation of foot to line of transmitted
        weight through leg, 61
    roentgenological, 64
    routine method for, 59
    shoe-study in, 64
    structural defects, 62
    toes, 62
    transverse arch, 61
Examining stand, **59**
Exercises, flexion and extension, 330
    foot adduction (standing), 334
        walking, 335
    heel stretching (sitting), 337
        standing, 338
    toe gripping, 332
    toe spreading, 331
Exostosis, operation for removal of, **225**
    x-ray of, **262**